About the

Sylvia Patterson is one of pop jc
Born in Perth, Scotland, she mo
twenty, to join *Smash Hits* as Stafi
for *NME*, *The Face*, *Glamour*, *Q*,
publications across the UK and US. Her first memoir, *I'm Not with the Band* (2016), was shortlisted for the Costa Biography Award, the Penderyn Music Book Prize, the NME Awards Book of the Year and won BBC Radio 1 DJ Annie Nightingale's Book of the Year. This is her second memoir.

Praise for *Same Old Girl*

'Inspired, impressive, unfailingly frank ... [a] thoroughly engaging, life-affirming book' *Mail on Sunday*

'Patterson brings much rackety humour to bear, despite the gravity of the subject ... Her book is a middle finger to cancer, a tribute to dogged survival' *Spectator*

'Reading *Same Old Girl* is to be reminded that there can still be laughter in the dark ... Patterson is one of the great comic writers of the last quarter century' *Herald*

'Unsparing but ultimately uplifting, every sentence cuts a caper even as it delivers a gruelling detail, or profound insight' *Mojo*

'Eye-watering, bone-shivering, soul-shaking and, yes, laugh-raising and spirit-lifting detail ... a relatable read by a phenomenal writer' *The Face*

'There's no mistaking the writing of Sylvia Patterson' *Sunday Times*

SAME OLD GIRL

SYLVIA PATTERSON

FLEET
2024

FLEET

First published in Great Britain in 2023 by Fleet
This paperback edition published in 2024 by Fleet

1 3 5 7 9 10 8 6 4 2

A CIP catalogue record for this book is available from the British Library.

ISBN 978-0-349-72746-2

Typeset in Caslon by M Rules
Printed and bound in Great Britain by Clays Ltd, Elcograf S.p.A.

Papers used by Fleet are from well-managed forests
and other responsible sources.

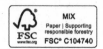

Fleet
An imprint of
Little, Brown Book Group
Carmelite House
50 Victoria Embankment
London EC4Y 0DZ

An Hachette UK Company
www.hachette.co.uk

www.littlebrown.co.uk

TO THE MIRACLE OF OUR NHS

CONTENTS

'Help me, Clarence. Get me back. Please, I wanna live again!'

George Bailey, *It's A Wonderful Life*

THE BEST DAYS OF OUR LIVES

24 November 2019.

'Here we ... here we ... here we fucking go!'

Aberdeen is going *berserk*. Fifteen thousand punters in the P&J Live arena are hollering their heads off as Gerry Cinnamon, a wee Glaswegian fellow with an acoustic guitar, plays his rousing folk-pop stunners. The full-capacity crowd, legs like pistons, are thumping the wooden floor, the jubilation equalling a raucous Celtic wedding knees-up, on Hogmanay. Scotland loves a party, a singsong and a communal comedy chant and here comes the Cinnamon signature, the sound of KC and the Sunshine Band's 1982 disco-pop thriller 'Give It Up', reworded for their national hero: 'Nah na na na na na na na na na *naaaah* ... Gerry Cinnamon ... Cinnamon! ... *Gerry Cinnamon* ...' The atmosphere, now, echoes the barnstorming lunacy of a rollicking World Darts final.

Ali is right beside me, where she's been so often throughout almost five decades of friendship, forty-nine years on from the five-year-olds who lived around the corner from each other in 'bonnie' Perth, central Scotland. Now fifty-four, we've freewheeled through a seventies childhood together, pounded garden paths on pogo sticks together, walked to school together, survived adolescence together, sheltered each other through parental booze problems together, discovered music together, enthusiastically negotiated sex, cider and cigarettes together, been on holiday together, moved to different countries not together and turned up on each other's doorsteps anyway (even the year she lived in Australia). On and on we've endured, our lives unfolding through all the silliness, pain, loss, hope, fear and joy of what it means to be an adult human being.

We've been music fanatics for ever, whether cackling at the idiocy of Queen's 'Bohemian Rhapsody' ('Bismilla! Nooo!') or roaring every word of The Eagles' 'Lyin' Eyes' ('I guess every form of refuge has its priiice') or pirouetting to Abba, a blonde (me) and a redhead (her) pretending we were the mighty Agnetha and Frieda. Until *Grease* was released in '78 and *everyone* pretended they were Bad Sandy in the leggings, with the fag.

And now here we are again, like teenagers again, singing and dancing and laughing and drinking, like we always did and always do, given a lot less than half the chance.

'This is the proper stuff!' blares Ali in my ear; she's always blaring in my ear, with the throaty guffaw of a woman with a flip-top head. Arms pumping overhead we're now roaring together the central line in Gerry Cinnamon's joyous 'Dark Days': 'These are the best days that you're ever gonna have!'

After post-gig drinks we fall into the same bed at a nearby hotel, she chortling as ever, me only pretending, really, that everything is quite this funny. Because I know, when I wake up, I have to tell her. That I think I'm going to die.

September 2019.

There's something wrong with my right nipple. I'm standing in the shower when I notice for the first time: it's deep red, weepy, scabby.

What the hell's that? That's weird. That's really weird. Hmm, must be the cheap sports bra I bought off Amazon, probably psoriasis, even though I've never had that. Typical, a comedy ailment, it's like being in an episode of Embarrassing Bodies . . .

Cursing Amazon and its cheapo 'bargains', I come up with a crafty ruse: a slither of Sudocrem on a circular makeup pad pressed to the nipple, held in place by a bra.

That should do it. Sudocrem is miraculous, and this weirdness will go away.

It doesn't go away. By early November the heebie-jeebies have arrived. So, I do what we all do when the heebie-jeebies turn up: I google it.

Oh no. OH NO.

A selection of strangers' red-raw nipples glisten out from my computer screen while my heartrate begins to climb. This is Paget's disease, and my weirdness looks exactly like this weirdness. I click on the trusty NHS website.

Paget's disease of the nipple, also known as Paget's disease of the breast, is a rare condition associated with breast cancer. It causes eczema-like changes to the skin of the nipple and the area of darker skin surrounding the nipple (areola). It's usually a sign of breast cancer in the tissue behind the nipple.

Oh dear God, I've got breast cancer. Er . . . I don't know that yet! Oh yes I do. Oh God, I've got breast cancer.

I scroll some more.

Around half of all women diagnosed with Paget's disease of the nipple have a lump behind the nipple. In nine out of ten cases this is an invasive breast cancer.

*Nine out of ten! I definitely *have* breast cancer!*

I've taken zero solace from the 'half of all women' statistic. I *know* I'm in the wrong half. All the liquid instantly drains from my mouth, heart now pounding, scrolling further down to where the treatments are listed, including mastectomy, chemotherapy, radiotherapy. I go onto my doctor's website and make an appointment. Next available: three weeks' time.

I could be dead by then!

The calendar on the kitchen wall, featuring scenic Scottish landscapes, now has the word 'Doc' written on the forthcoming appointment day, while I attempt to forget about it, for now. Which is impossible. My partner of almost two decades, Simon, I decide, doesn't need to know. He'll only worry. Neither of us should worry until there's something to worry about. A week later he notices 'Doc' on the calendar.

'What's this for?'

'Er, there's something wrong with my nipple. Embarrassingly enough. It might be nothing. I don't know. But I'll know soon.'

His already expansive pale blue eyes extend to the size of breadbins. 'What d'you mean, "Wrong with it?"'

'It's probably just a skin thing. Don't worry!'

I'm worried. Waves of fear, in fact, wash in and out of my mind every day for three weeks as if pulled by the eternal tide. My brain won't stop thinking about Gavin, my friend since the late eighties, who I worked with on soaraway pop bible S*mash Hits*. He married my other *Smash Hits* buddy, Leesa, and I was one of the bridesmaids at their wedding in 2008. They had their first child in 2012 and in 2013 Gavin was diagnosed with pancreatic cancer, given one year to live and died in 2014, aged forty-four. We'd all watched this handsome, hilarious, physically robust man (a non-smoking, teetotal marathon runner by then) shrink to a skeletal spectre while making jokes, still, on Facebook. His legs were skinnier, he quipped, than Mo Farah's. 'They're Less Farah.' Everyone loved Gavin. Bastard cancer.

I've got cancer, I know it. What if it's really bad? What if it's spread? What if I'm told, like Gavin, I've got one year to live? There's no reason why that can't happen to me, no reason at all. Why me? Why not? Oh, please don't let me die, not yet, I'm not finished! Yes, and with a two-year-old son and a wife, neither was Gavin. Shut up, brain, and deal with it when you have to!

I have flashbacks of shopping in Tesco in that shocking death year of 2014, when life felt so suddenly fragile: waiting in line for the self-service till, the instructional stand-up queue sign, I was certain, was pointedly telling me something: 'YOU'RE NEXT'.

Appointment day. The GP, a stranger, as is often the way in London, surveys the nipple and examines the breast, strong fingers nudging into the mounds and around the folds.

'I can't feel any lumps,' she notes, frankly, 'but I'll send you for a mammogram anyway. They'll be looking for cancer but that doesn't mean this is cancer, OK?'

20 November, 2019.

Mammograms aren't hugely painful but they're certainly unpleasant. One of the lovely, efficient radiographers motions me towards the edge of a bulky machine a bit like a 1950s hooded hairdryer, with two scanner plates jutting outwards in the middle, picks up my right bosom as if it's a fleshy flap on a hinge and places it directly onto the bottom plate. She guides me further forward, until as much flesh as possible is splayed onto the plate and turns a wheel that makes the scanner descend, digging uncomfortably into the upper ribs. My breast is now in a vice, flattened, pulled out from my body like a beige, squashed jellyfish. The same then happens sideways – the machine turned 180 degrees, plates narrowing in from the sides – the breast now reduced to a cylinder of fat and tissue where an orb of pleasure once was. I put my clothes back on and tears spring into my eyes. I've had mammograms before, but this time feels so different. Because this time isn't routine. I look towards the radiographer observing her computer, a black screen showing the milky mosaic of the inside of my right breast. She sees me staring, looks up and speaks.

'It's a lot to take in.'

I'm startled, silent, thoughts thundering through my mind.

What is? I haven't been told anything yet. But I know that terminology. That's what nurses and doctors say when you're diagnosed with a life-threatening disease. If not a terminal one!

She could see what was there and I couldn't. She knew and I didn't.

Except I did, now.

I'm sent to see a consultant who tells me there's 'something there' but I'll have to wait for official results. I'm shaking, heart thumping.

'So ... it might not be cancer?'

'It might not be. But if it is, don't worry, it could be manageable. And you're in the process now.'

I'm in the process now. The process! I know that terminology, too. That also means I've got cancer. He knows. Of course he knows. I have cancer. And maybe it's not *manageable! I've had no tests done for a spread to anywhere else. But now I know I definitely have cancer.*

Four days later in Aberdeen, Ali is the first person I'm planning to tell about my imminent death, beyond Simon – who's currently in London, planning my funeral in his head. I've had no parents since the age of thirty-nine so they, at least, don't have to deal with this. I haven't yet told my sisters, or my other friends, or Simon's parents. Ali will be first to know – not by design, but simply timing: in late 2019 I'm still a music journalist, still working for *Q* magazine and on assignment – to interview Gerry Cinnamon and see him play live in Aberdeen. Ali lives sixteen miles away in Stonehaven, so it was all the excuse I needed: I'd invite her along, for a laugh, and she could stay in my hotel room.

For four days I've been inwardly churning with fear, a constant tension awaiting screening results which will tell me how long I have left to live. It might not be very long. I've been thinking about death constantly, really thinking about death, in a way you don't until you're facing it. What is it, ultimately, that we're all so very afraid of?

I don't think we fear The Moment of Death itself. Most of us will have a deathbed, either in hospital, a hospice or at home. I know from seeing the death of both my parents up close, in hospital, that end-of-life care is overwhelmingly morphine-assisted, a rainbow-coloured dreamscape of semi-consciousness and shallow breathing until your breath simply stops. And that's it. It's what nurses and doctors mean by 'making-someone-comfortable'.

I don't think we fear the pain involved or debilitating physical circumstances, possibly living horribly compromised for years, because people endure these traumas with heroic amounts of grace, good humour and unfeasible positivity everywhere you look.

No. It's the blackout. The void. The space where you once were no longer with you in it, while everyone and everything else you've ever known and loved carries on regardless. It's the turning into a memory. It's so much more than a fleeting FOMO, the missing out on the good times, it's the missing out on all that future life, the one with the young people in it, with everyone growing old. Which is beyond fear into a canyon-deep chasm of sadness. A primal howl of, 'Noooooooo!' It's the colossal *swizz* of it all. And the pulverising wrecking ball which pounds into your gut when you think you're about to die is the most profound version of missing out that it's possible to feel. We only fear death, I guess, because we love life so much.

But it's also – and it might be the greater of the two – the fear of what will happen to the people you love when you're gone, depending on the circumstances, on how much they depend on you. Or those who simply need and want you to stay alive, for as long as they're alive (as unlikely as that often is, unless you die at exactly the same time, in surely tragic circumstances). Grief, as the saying goes, truly *is* the price of love.

'I thought, My God, my dad's gonna die of a heart attack.' So confided Kylie Minogue back in 2007, two years after the breast cancer diagnosis she was convinced would kill her, aged thirty-six. 'So much stress on the whole family,' she added, 'that was very painful.'

I've been a music journalist since teenhood; from rookie beginnings in Dundee at the fabled DC Thomson publishing empire, to joining *Smash Hits* pop gazette at twenty in early 1986. I've rollicked through print music journalism ever since, as its relevance, purpose and presence began fading through the decades, as technology changed everything, to its near obsolescence as a cultural force today. The solo artist I've interviewed more times than any other is pop's effervescent Tinker Bell: Kylie, from her toothsome *Smash Hits* days onwards, through *Sky* magazine, *NME* and *Q*, right up until 2019, months before Covid capsized the global music industry. Back in 2007, aged thirty-nine, she said she absolutely believed she would die, just as I will on a wintry night in Aberdeen twelve years later.

'Was I thinking, That's it, I'm going to fall off my perch? Oh yes. Yeah, yeah, yeah,' she nodded, vigorously. 'I was really scared. Upset. Angry. But comfort comes wherever you choose to find it. The letters I got from kids who just knew I was sick. They were like, "We're sorry you have to see the doctors and we don't want them to put needles in you. And you're the best singer in the world!" It was just so genuine.

'But even though I'm cancer-free, I have memories every day of it,' she noted. 'You're physically and mentally scarred, but that doesn't stop you getting on with what becomes the new normal. Of course, my heart goes out to anyone in that situation; health problems affect everybody. But it was the first time I'd experienced anything to that degree. Very traumatic. And I came out of it thinking, Wow, that was a great lesson in humanity; that's what I took from it. Meeting people I would never have met. That part was amazing.'

I'd wondered that year what Kylie thought her purpose was, as a creative entity. 'Sparkle, joy, dreams, I think that's my purpose,' she decided. By 2019 she'd changed her mind. 'I would say something different now,' she mused. 'I would say: "Light." Light with reflection. A reflection of oneself? And light doesn't come without dark. So, if I can represent sparkle, shimmer, shine, I think what it also says is "Hope". Hope in the dark. Hope in what we're all trying to get through. Rising above.'

So, at the end of 2019, it was Kylie Minogue of all people, the sometime unknowable pop hologram, who was the one public figure bringing me bolstering anecdotal evidence, comfort and indeed hope. Even if, right now, in Aberdeen, lying wide awake in a hotel bed, I'm planning to tell my oldest pal, just as Kylie believed, that I'm about to fall off my perch.

2

DREAMS OF CHILDREN

We're ten years old, me 'n' Ali, sitting face to face on an industrial stone wall and playing cards, as the train from Perth to Dundee thrillingly thunders by, two feet away from our faces. It's one of our favourite places to go, four metres above ground between the walkway and the railway track of Perth's Tay Viaduct, wind blowing the hair backwards on we blissfully naive children. A fully grown man approaches one day, a man we'll soon decide has a 'funny jaw'. He asks if we'd like to go with him to the nearby Norie-Miller Walk, a scenic riverside stroll, 'to pick daffodils'. We look at each other, stifling giggles, ignore him and get back to our cards. He wanders away. Our parents have no idea where we are. We're simply 'out', together, and that's good enough for them.

Perth, 1975 and we were never in. Out was where the larks were, all the mirth and the malarkey, forever on bikes, spacehoppers or cavorting around the two parks of Perth known, for reasons I've never unearthed, as 'Inches': the North Inch and, inevitably, the South Inch. The North Inch was where a large domed building was opened in 1968, a landed spaceship known as Bell's Sports Centre and surely the only sporting facility ever to be named after a whisky baron (Arthur Kinmond Bell, fiscally generous local philanthropist and peddler of blended Bell's, the worst whisky in the world).

Me 'n' Ali from around the corner had two other best pals we'd grown up with since the age of five (remaining entwined in each other's lives to this day). Evelyn (Ev), from around-three-corners, the garden of her family home stretching, handily, onto the North Inch. She was, perhaps, the most level-headed among us, a can-do kind of person who'd take charge of outdoors 'den' building, who loved both brawny rugby and campy dressing up (and kept a well-stocked dressing-up box).

And Jill who lived around, say, twenty corners, on a housing estate towards the north, the tomboy of the crew, whose party trick was squirting jets of water through her charmingly gappy teeth (especially at boys, as adolescence arrived). We are The Four of Us. The North Inch became our communal playground, where rounders was played, bikes were fallen off and boys would one day be snogged.

It was me 'n' Ali, though, who were out the most, the others' parents more vigilant than ours (applying something alien to us called 'rules'). When we weren't out on the Inches we were up Buckie Braes, a local hillside woodland where we swung from tree branches by perilously fraying ropes. Once, Ali dramatically lost her grip with a terrifying shriek, thumping onto her spine mere inches from a spikey stake of tree stump. In all weathers we'd visit The Hermitage, a stunning forest walk in nearby Dunkeld, its unique botanicals so vividly green, russet and purple, you'd expect goblins to appear on the mossy, velvety boulders.

We spent so much time together because our family life was complicated, in different ways. Ali was what we called in those supposedly carefree days 'a latchkey kid', an only child whose mum, a cook, worked mostly until 1.30 a.m. at the local hospital. It was where she first met my mum, a psychiatric nurse, and through them we were introduced. Ali's dad, therefore, was free to spend nights with his pals in the pubs and social clubs of Perth, as long as Ali was at mine, which she usually was, seeing as the alternative was home alone. And when we weren't at mine, we were larking around Bell's, or wandering 'downtown' where we'd loiter in the Wimpy with a Coke Float, Banana Split or towering Knickerbocker Glory.

My parents, meanwhile, had two generations of kids: Billy, Ronnie and Liz were baby boomers born in the late forties and early fifties and myself and sister Jackie, born early-to-mid-sixties, which makes me seventeen years younger than the eldest. Billy and Liz had long left home by the time I was five while Jackie, exactly four years older to the day, had her own buddies (and boyfriends). She'd try out makeup looks on her little sister and ever-present pal, experimental plasterings in neon-blue eyeshadow, lip gloss and powder, before she headed out on a Saturday night. Then we'd rummage through her mid-seventies wardrobe, dress up in her cheesecloth shirts, flares and platform shoes and dance around the twin bedroom me 'n' Jackie shared, 'freaking out' to Abba. Feeling particularly brave (foolish) one Saturday night, we each wore one of Jackie's bras, stuffed with socks, and teetered around the nearby and notoriously shady housing estate.

My other sibling at home was Ronnie, a Down's syndrome person and the gentlest soul I'd ever know. Most evenings he'd recline in his living-room armchair, me 'n' Ali hiding behind, encouraging him to 'scare' us by flailing his arms behind the chair, which we all found hugely amusing, especially when the Curly Wurly stashed up his cardigan sleeve plummeted to the floor.

My dad had a garage-sized shed that provided hours of jocular japes, a scrap merchant's junkyard packed with blade-heavy tools and overhead hanging hoses, where we'd black out the windows with blankets and play blind hide 'n' seek. We called this game, to make it extra funny, 'Man in the Dark'.

And we danced, constantly. Scotland is a dancing kind of country, and growing up there, particularly in the seventies, you were encouraged to learn the ancient customs. From the age of ten to thirteen, every Monday night, we'd dutifully arrive in a small, draughty church hall to waft our limbs to the Highland Fling in embroidered white blouses, kilts a-swing, like girly saps on a tartan tin of all-butter Crawford's shortbread. But it was pop culture which formed us, freeing us from the tartan traditions, two early teenagers fortunate enough to be this exact age, at this exact time, when Abba and the Bee Gees were the biggest pop bands on Earth; obsessive devotees who saw both *Abba: The Movie* and *Saturday Night Fever* at 'the pictures', *twice*.

When *Grease* was released in '78 we raised the obsessional bar, not only seeing it *five* times at the pictures, but enrolling in 'John Travolta Dancing Classes' in yet another small church hall, where twelve-to-thirteen-year-old girls were taught the synchronised routines to both the *Grease* soundtrack and Travolta's fabled *Fever* moves. We'd point to the sky, point to the floor, squealing every word to every song, with extra gusto, naturally, for 'Stayin' Alive', with the wings of heaven on our shoes, dancing men who just could not lose.

By early '79, as the post-punk uprising ricocheted out of the radio, up the charts and into our living rooms through *Top of the Pops*, as the booze, cigarettes, pubs and clubs shimmered on the horizon of full-blown adolescence, we still managed to remain kids. At just turned fourteen we were bounding around our living rooms to the hits of irresistibly anthemic Scotsmen The Skids, 'Masquerade! Masquerade!', high-kicking behind the couch in an approximation of an ecstatic punk-rock can-can. We found everything funny. Maybe because so much, elsewhere, wasn't funny.

Through the 1970s my mum had become a frightening presence at home, an increasingly volatile alcoholic I no longer recognised as Mum, a belligerent, alien forcefield who lived behind a closed living-room door, where the shouting happened, where me 'n'

Ali never ventured (nor Jackie or Ronnie) and where the sadness lived for my funny, gentle father. No wonder we were always together, me and the latchkey kid, bouncing to the music, lost in its infinite freedom.

I guess we relied on each other without realising it, two kids growing up in identical geographical coordinates, exactly the same age, with a similar sense of humour and heightened appreciation of silliness, absurdism, escapism and music. There were The Four Of Us, always, and there always will be. But far more than us, Ev and Jill were bound by time constraints, discipline and boundaries. Me 'n' Ali were the ones without a steady anchor, without a guiding compass, so we gravitated towards each other's free-floating lives, finding continuity, safety and companionship, forever dancing, laughing, after the same rainbow's end. And fifty-odd years later she's still there. Waitin' round the bend.

My huckleberry friend.

3

ALBATROSS

25 November 2019, Hotel Moxy, Aberdeen.

We wake up, me 'n' Ali, a pair of fifty-four-year-olds still thrilled over our big night out with the Arena-sized Glaswegian busker. On and on we burble about how rollicking Cinnamon was and I play her the song he doesn't play live any more, which I know she'll love, about Scottish independence. It's called 'Hope Over Fear'. I have a shower. She has a shower. We put our clothes on. We put our makeup on together, like we've been doing for forty years.

'I've got something to tell you.'

'Oh? Oh, OK.'

'I'm having tests done for breast cancer.'

Silence. Starey eyes.

'And I'm pretty sure I've got it. I fact I *know* I've got it. But I don't how bad it is yet.'

'Oh. Oh wow.'

She comes towards me like she always does, her arms straight out to the sides like an albatross in flight. She throws them around me and I breathe in the unmistakeable smell of her, an Estée Lauder perfume called 'Youth Dew' she's been wearing for decades. I burst into tears. Her eyes brim. She says it again.

'Oh wow.'

We disentangle, look straight into each other's moist green eyes and she sits down on the double bed.

'Oh wow. Oh wow. *Oh wow.*'

'I'll know how bad it is in a couple of weeks.'

She pauses.

'Don't you dare.'

Ali has worked for the NHS since the 1980s and in late 2019 is the Senior Charge Nurse in a stroke rehabilitation ward in Aberdeen. She has, therefore, an insider's perspective. She now tells me not only what I need to hear but the truth as she knows it. It's not like the seventies any more, she assures, or even the eighties or nineties. There are incredibly effective treatments now, targeted chemotherapies, if you must have a breast off *fuck it*, and they do reconstructions as routine now, anyway. I would be all right, millions upon millions of women across the planet survive this thing every year, for decades. *I would be all right.*

She drives us through heavy, east-coast rain to her home in Stonehaven and I mention *Beaches*, the 1989 movie where two lifelong friends, a showgirl and a lawyer, face the fatal illness of one of them, together. It's usually Ali who mentions it first, a gallows-humour quip about some rum scenario we'll doubtless face in the future. And now the future has turned up early. I weep every time I hear Bette Midler sing the theme tune, 'Wind Beneath My Wings', with its vaguely fitting lyrics, about the showbiz one with all the glory, the lawyer with all the strength. We were never each other's heroes, never wanted to be each other, we were equals and opposites, with almost comically contrasting personalities, lifestyles, jobs and domestic set-ups but the lyrics, nonetheless, destroy me every time: Midler flies higher than an eagle, 'for you are the wind beneath my wings'.

Ali was still driving through November rain when she glanced over.

'I always thought it would be me.'

'Did you?'

'Yes. But you'll be all right. *You'll be all right.* It's not gonny be *Beaches.*'

'Not yet?'

'Not yet.'

We're both hungover when she drives me to Aberdeen airport at 5.30 a.m. the following morning for the flight back to London, on her way to work at the hospital. The roads are eerily quiet, sparkling with overnight rain, the occasional delivery van a ghostly apparition scooshing through the darkness of a Scottish winter before dawn. No, I never wanted to be Ali all right, this was a normal working day for her, while I'd spent decades carousing around London and much of the planet living the irresponsible bedlam-shaped dream of music journalism, a job now as antiquated as working in a sixties' typing pool. And Ali, she'd told me many times, even back-in-the-day when the music press still thrived, could never have tolerated the financial chaos of my insecure freelance life.

She pulls up just beyond an airport roundabout, tells me again I'll be all right and to keep her constantly updated. We wave goodbye as she drives out of sight and I trundle my wheelie case into a deserted Aberdeen airport, check in and go through security. I'm starving. A café is serving already, an open-plan bistro looking onto WH Smiths where fairy lights weakly twinkle in the stark overhead lighting, piles of selection boxes towering as high as Scottish mountains. I order at the counter: coffee, sparkling water, £6.95 worth of avocado on toast (outrageous) and sit with the drinks at a table, waiting for the posho toast. Staring over at the Christmas lights, I'm contemplating the contents of the selection boxes, featuring much of the confectionery me 'n' Ali would've found in our Christmas stocking (a pillowcase) all the way through the seventies: Crunchie, Mars Bar, Topic (a hazelnut in every bite). Music is piping quietly through the café. For all the talk from both of us of how I'd be all right, I didn't know if I *would* be all right, at all. How could I? Life has taught me never to presume. Presumption, as someone wise once told me, is the mother of all fuck-ups. I was heading back to London to find out, realistically, how long I had to live. I'd been a teenage goth back in the early eighties, a vision of fright-wigged intensity who always felt somehow *doomed*. And the miserable bastard, evidently, lurked inside me still.

This really might be my last Christmas. Please don't let this be my last Christmas. I really hope they don't play 'Last Christmas'. But if it is, can I complain, really? I'm ancient now, even though I feel thirty-five and have done for twenty years. And I've had a good life, haven't I? I haven't wasted it, have I? It's been ... mental. I always wanted things to be mental. Oh God, I hope this isn't the price for all that mental – all those fags and booze and spliffs and more fags. And I'm still addicted to nicotine. I can't live without my vape, I've been addicted to nicotine for the 'best' part of forty years. But millions of people get breast cancer – a spectrum of cancers – who've never smoked one snout in their life. Including toddlers! So stop beating yourself up! Shut up, shut up, shut up ...

Then, an unmistakable guitar ping. The opening notes of The Eagles' 'Lyin' Eyes'. My avocado on toast arrives. I ignore the mossy mash-up and listen to the lyrics I've loved since I was ten years old, especially that killer line about forms of refuge having their price. An involuntarily chin-wobble. It's a line which has meant something to me for ever, through all those refuges I'd escaped to throughout the decades, whether some crazy boy, alcohol, relentless work or everything music can be and do at its most emotionally profound. I was someone who'd made music their *life*.

Another line cuts through, the one about how your new life didn't change things.

My throat contracts, a hard swallow attempts to keep it open, to keep me breathing.

'You're still the same old girl you used to be ...'

Like a rupture in the Earth's crust, the lyric breaks me open, a tsunami of emotion roars through my ears, face flushing radioactive crimson. I *wasn't* the same old girl I used to be. I was someone else now. *Something* else. I was about to become a very ill person. Very possibly someone who was living through the last few years of their life. This thing would change me for ever. Wouldn't it? How couldn't it? I knew it. *I just knew it.* My luck had run out. And I wasn't even particularly lucky. I wouldn't make it to be old, after all. Then, The Fear.

Oh God, what will happen to Simon? He can't afford to live in our flat on his own. We've no life insurance between us, because we're juvenile, reality-dodging idiots. If I die, my beloved sister Jackie won't cope. She's in the middle of a divorce after nearly forty years of marriage, for a start. What about my lovely wee niece ... and nephew ... and all my lifelong pals, they don't deserve this nonsense cluttering up their lives.

I felt so ... *robbed.* Fifty-four, really, wasn't old. I felt crumpled up and tiny, like a car crushed in an industrial compactor, wheels pinged off, my whole life now condensed into a tiny cube of memory for anyone who had ever cared. It was the worst instance of a thousand instances over the course of our lives that had caused me 'n' Ali to have a catchphrase: 'Swizzed again!'

Band Aid's 'Do They Know It's Christmas' pipes through the café. 'Tonight thank God it's them, instead of yoooooo!' yodels Bono. For some people back in Ethiopia in 1984, they didn't reach *four*, never mind fifty-four.

Stop yer blubbin', Patterson!

I stop. Eat the smashed avocado on toast. And head home to whatever the future holds. For however long the future will last.

Here we, here we, here we fucking go ...

4

UNCOMFORTABLY NUMB

I'm on a bus with Simon, in silence, rolling through streets we've both bussed, walked, taxied and stumbled through for almost fifteen years, from our north London neighbourhood of Hornsey, through boho Crouch End, up towards the Northern Hospital. These streets could not be more familiar and yet now they're alien, distorted as if through a gauze, somehow fictional roads in the film of someone else's life. It's as if they're reflected in a pond and, should my hand reach out and touch them through an open window, they would disappear in outwardly circling ripples of illusion. Nothing feels real. What's that all about? Google knows.

Derealisation.

Derealisation is an alteration in the perception of the external world, causing sufferers to perceive it as unreal, distant, distorted or falsified. Other symptoms include feeling as if one's environment is lacking in spontaneity, emotional colouring and depth. It is a dissociative symptom that may appear in moments of severe stress.

I'm clutching Simon's knee. We clutch at things – ourselves, our partners, our kids, random objects, cups of tea – for comfort, but how is someone's *knee* supposed to help you? Especially Simon's left knee, which is half the size of his 'good' right knee, being someone born with a club foot (*talipes equinovarus*), which not only skews his foot into a hoof shape but renders his lower leg, from the knee down, a spindle. But this is the knee I need on this frosty late November morning when we're both about to find out how long I have to live.

The bus trundles on and random flashbacks appear of good times, back to the whirling jamboree of the 1990s and a conversation I once had with Pulp's angle-poise-lamp-limbed frontman Jarvis Cocker. In 1995 I gave him the opportunity to write his own headstone epitaph, for *Sky* magazine, in those sepia-tinted days when magazine culture not only existed but flourished, and was funny, and mattered.

'I'll have to have a piss while I think about that,' he chirped, heading to a nearby loo where he began shouting, with the door wide open. '"Here lies Jarvis Cocker, now thinner than ever",' he quipped, padding back to his seat. 'I always wanted to have a video camera in me coffin. And have the gravestone with a TV screen on it so people could see me rotting away. I think it's good to see a dead body. When me granddad died, we had the coffin open in the house. It's not pleasant, but at least it makes you realise they're really dead. You're always going to feel sorry that someone dies, but when you realise they're actually gone you can get on with things. People shouldn't feel sorry for you because you're dead: you're just dead, aren't you? You're not suffering anything. People might just miss you a bit, that's all.'

I clutch Simon's knee all the tighter.

Walking into the consultant surgeon's room we're still in silence, now seated side by side in front of a desk. My surgeon is – I think still unusually – a woman, an efficient, frank, warm-eyed consultant called Ms Jana, who sits before us with her large computer screen showing that milky mosaic of my right breast. She goes straight into diagnosis, so speedily I barely hear it. She doesn't say, 'You have cancer,' but I definitely hear, as she points at the screen, 'and this is your tumour,' something about an area of pre-cancerous cells and something about 'treatable' which is, I already know, the only word you really need to hear. On hearing 'treatable' I feel an electric jolt of euphoria, now so deliriously optimistic I'm inventing my own prognosis, which pinballs through my head, blocking out everything else the expert is trying to tell me.

If it hasn't spread there'll be surgery in a few weeks, breast off at worst – who cares as long as I'm alive? – a bit of radiotherapy and by early spring I'll be cartwheeling round Ally Pally Park, blubbing at the sound of woodpeckers, as usual. Won't I?

Not so fast, old girl. Biopsies and scans are still needed, I'm now hearing, to determine if the cancer has spread or not and, therefore, if I'm likely to stay alive or not. She sets up a treatment plan appointment with an oncologist, a Dr Badger, who I like the comedy sound of already in my suddenly comedy-free life.

Two breast-care nurses, Renée and Keren, take us into a side-room where we're given a tower of booklets and leaflets on all aspects of breast cancer, the pair of us seated, dumbstruck, while a foreign language of information buries us alive. Outside the hospital, bewildered, shocked at the sudden realness of it all, I break down, sobbing in the street. All I know for certain is appointments for several biopsies have been made, and I've no idea what having a biopsy even entails.

Lying on a day-patient table in the Northern, breasts exposed to a roomful of strangers, a bustling man bears down on me with an implement as alarming as a shark hunter's harpoon. 'Sharp scratch,' he warns and plunges the needle in so deeply, so painfully, I let loose an involuntary shriek and jackknife halfway off the table.

'Sorry, sorry!' I'm squalling, 'I wasn't expecting that!'

I don't know what I was expecting, exactly (a barely there

pinprick with a thumb tack?) but this needs to be done twice, so I'm pumped with what seems to be enough adrenalin-infused anaesthetic to keep a horse alive through a four-leg amputation. This induces hand-shake tremors so violent I feel like a particularly unfortunate eighty-two-year-old Parkinson's patient already.

The following day, while lying on another table, breasts exposed once more, Ms Jana, having administered a far less drama-inducing anaesthetic, looms over me with a glinting scalpel and announces, 'I don't like the look of this.' Neither do I, frankly, as the scalpel in her hand descends and slices into my right nipple, a small but significant part of which is dropped into a jar and placed on a medical tray, to be carted off on its lonesome journey to the lab. I should 'prepare', she tells me, 'for a mastectomy, but we'll see', pending all the results to come.

A week later Ms Jana sits again at her desk. The tumour, she explains, is a rapid grower, 'aggressive', so I'll need chemotherapy imminently and for the next six months, to shrink the tumour and aid surgical success. Followed by radiotherapy. And probably a full mastectomy. Just the one breast off, mind. My initial overwhelming thought is, You can take an arm and a leg while you're at it, as long as I stay alive. I even suggest having the other one off at the same time, because not only would that be less hideous, there'd be nowhere for anything to grow in the other, possibly predatory, breast. But that's not, I'm told, how cancer works. Any cancer you have, if it's going to grow again, could grow anywhere throughout the body, in any of your organs, bones, skin, head, all of it. And no one in the NHS ever wants to amputate a healthy part of anyone's body. So I simply accept it, as part of 'the process' which can keep me alive.

My personal, bespoke, especially-for-you type of breast cancer is HER2 Positive (written HER2+), which sounds like a troubled trans woman's self-empowerment workshop but stands for the significantly less motivational human epidermal growth factor receptor 2. It's a protein, the presence of which cheerleads the tumour into Miracle-Gro abundance, meaning highly aggressive, Grade 3 cancer cells. It's the kind of cancer both Kylie and Jennifer Saunders had, so at least I'm in excellent company. The good news is the biopsy they took of my lymph nodes, near the underarm, is clear. There's no guarantee it hasn't spread anywhere else but until they know otherwise, this cancer remains 'treatable' and indeed 'manageable'.

'So don't worry too much,' says the gracious Ms Jana, 'we've caught it early.'

Miraculously, the dodgy nipple almost certainly saved my life. It *was* Paget's disease, a separate kind of cancer, the warning flare that made me make the initial appointment, when no one, not me, nor the fondling local GP, could detect another tumour growing, rapidly, at the base of my right breast. So I was *very* fortunate, after all. But there are still more tests to come, for 'mets', the metastatic cancer cell spread which means a Stage 4 diagnosis and (predominantly) certain death.

The most common sites for breast cancer mets are bone, brain, liver and lung. I absorb this information knowing I have, over the decades, smoked what could well be *hundreds of thousands* of cigarettes. My inner teenage goth embalms me in a cocoon of numbness, a coping mechanism in part but, really, I'm saving all the anxiety for when there's something to be anxious about. I know I've been lucky so far. But I'm used to my luck running out. I've never felt particularly lucky, ever, there's always been too much chaos. I don't feel *all* that lucky right now.

We head back home and for the next three weeks I attempt to convince myself I'm not about to die. But I absolutely believe I am. And the scans to come will prove it. *I just know it.*

5

GHOST IN THE MACHINE

While waiting to hear from the biopsy results whether I'm about to die or not, I meet my oncologist for the first time. Disappointingly, she is not Dr Badger, as I'd misheard, but Dr Bridger, who does not disappoint at all; she is the definition of steadfast, professional and knowledgeable. The fact I now have an oncologist is preposterous to me. I don't think I've ever said 'oncologist' out loud before, a clumsy word which makes your tongue contort at the back of your teeth, a word which stems from the Greek root *'onkos'*, meaning 'mass', as in 'mass of toxic cells'. *Brrrrr.* She is smartly dressed in a crisp shirt and pencil skirt, very slim, blonde hair in an efficient ponytail and holding an old-school pencil, hovering over a blank sheet of unlined A4 paper. She's detailing my treatment plan while *drawing* my treatment plan, a roughly sketched human cell, with lines poking outwards attached to the word HER2, decorated with various alarming words, like 'oestrogen-blocking treatment', 'Letrozole', 'five years'.

Five years? How ill am I exactly!? I don't feel ill at all. Oestrogen blocking? Don't I need my oestrogen for all that ... womanly stuff?

She carries on writing, something about 'bone infusions', every six months for three years, to stop the onset of chemo-related osteoporosis.

Fabulous. So now, for someone described as a 'geezer bird' back in the nineties, I'm not only going be even more of a bloke than I am already but a ninety-five-year-old bloke with rickets.

Chemotherapy, she confirms, will make my hair fall out and, just as I'm contemplating what kind of glamorous drag queen's wig might suit me best, she mentions something called the cold cap. This will freeze my scalp, and therefore hair follicles, which stops at least some falling out. Only if you can tolerate, mind, having your head frozen for the three-hour chemo section of up to eight hours of treatment (depending on other 'infusions' you might need).

'We've had some very successful outcomes with hair,' she notes and adds, possibly in hope rather than expectation, 'and some people sail through chemo.'

I'm not going to sail through chemo. I'm not the sort of person who sails through anything. I'm far more likely to capsize my canoe in the first puddle you'd normally see a toddler gleefully jumping up and down in.

She wonders, casually, if I've ever smoked? I have smoked. I have smoked a lot. All kinds of cigarettes. The ones in packets. Roll-ups, which I'd particularly loved: skilfully hand-fashioned snouts swathed in liquorice cigarette papers which made them extra-delicious. Marijuana spliffs which, alongside the physical damage they caused, also made me mentally ill. The spectrum of ever-evolving vapes since 1997, between the real cigarettes, which I was always trying to give up. Today, I haven't smoked real tobacco for years but have no intention of giving up my beloved vape. I can't imagine life without it, the pleasure it brings is abundant.

Slender fingers rattle on clunky computer keys as she makes appointments for several vital scans which will determine if this thing has spread throughout my body. If it has, I will be officially doomed. I'm booked in for an MRI scan, CT scan, bone scan and an echo heart scan (or echocardiogram) because chemotherapy can badly damage the heart, which will be monitored throughout the treatment. The first three will happen on the same day, 19 December. Merry Christmas!

When you suddenly have a life-threatening illness and you're always going to hospital, you must immediately become fantastically organised. On the day of my three scans, I'm following a precisely scheduled itinerary:

7.00 a.m. Up! Take banana and pre-made cheese 'n' tom roll. Pack gift stuff to wrap and card. (It's Simon's birthday in two days' time and this is my only opportunity to wrap his present and write his card in secret.)

7.45 a.m. Leave house. Breakfast banana on bus.

8.45 a.m. MRI scan. Comfy clothes. Level three, imaging dept., Northern Hospital.

11.15 a.m. Nuclear medicine dept., level three. Bone scan injection tracer.

12.45 p.m. CT scan contrast drink, level three, imaging dept.

1.45 p.m. CT scan.

2.30-ish Lunch, drink plenty of water.

3.00 p.m. Bone scanner, nuclear medicine dept, level three.

4.30 p.m. Sheila Roberts, re: financial help in Macmillan Pod, foyer.

Each of my scans is a lifetime's first and I've no idea what to expect, just doing what I'm told to do in my regulation hospital gown, the billowingly shapeless white one with the blue diamond motif, my clothes piled on a plastic chair.

The MRI scan is mind-blowingly peculiar and unexpectedly gruelling.

The machine itself looks like a huge, white, cylindrical coffin which you slide all the way into. Lying face down on the movable bed, my two breasts dangle like exhausted udders into two, specially moulded, bosom-shaped holes. There is no dignity in this 'lark' and humiliation, already, has become a way of life. A radiologist tells me a) I must keep as still as possible for the next forty minutes and b) the noises will be LOUD. She positions a pair of bulky headphones around my head, at a wonky angle, as festive tunes from Heart FM come tinkling, tinnily, in the vague direction of my ears. Absolutely none of which can drown out the sonic booms now blasting through my head, as if robots are beaming industrial hazard signals straight into my violently vibrating eardrums. The sound, BEE-BOO-BEE-BOO-BOO-BOO-BOO-BEE-BOO-BEE-BOO-BEE, morphs into a sick joke, sounding like the repeated word 'booby' ... 'booby, booby, *booo-beeeee* ...' The whole universe is now surely having a laugh, as Heart FM vies for my bludgeoned attention via the merry jauntiness of Chris Rea's 'Driving Home for Christmas'.

The CT scan, by comparison, is a friendly tickle from a giant, ceramic Polo mint, lying atop a smooth, soundless bed, scooshing slowly in and out of the huge, circular scanner ring. No humiliation ensues, even if the contrast drink I'd downed beforehand, a dye which helps highlight what they're looking for – i.e. death – comes with warnings of nausea, vomiting, headache, itching, flushing and hives (all of which I'm spared).

Soon, I'm striding into the excitingly titled nuclear medicine department for the bone scan, my body now radioactive from an injection tracer, a liquid delivered intravenously through a thin tube attached to a needle now lodged in a vein in the back of my hand, a tube known as a cannula. Accompanying instructions demand no hugging of any children for the next six hours lest they become radioactive versions of the Ready Brek kids from the ads in the 1980s. Once more donning the regulation gown I'm positioned flat on my back on a medical bed and once more told to remain completely still. It's possible, in here, to be objective, to marvel at not only the sci-fi technology at work – large white panels of techno wizardry circling around your body – but your own actual skeleton, in fluorescent white, glowing at you from a screen.

Blimey, my spine is remarkably straight. Hang on ... what's that!?

I'm staring at a radioactive white light beaming like a solar flare from deep within my pelvis. This is what's known as a 'hot spot', indicating something sinister. A flood of terror flushes around my veins. I've had an on-off pain in that pelvic area for years *and done absolutely nothing about it*, convinced it was some wear and tear niggle, the kind you pick up in your fifties. Now? I *know* I have bone cancer, this thing has clearly spread, my stomach plummets to the floor, I am *definitely doomed*. The scan complete, I slide off the table and look one last time at the screen bearing my soon-to-be-dust skeleton. I stare even harder. There, in my pelvic area, is not only the hot-spot bone cancer explosion but – right in the middle – a large, solid-white pear-shape lying on its side. I blurt out to the radiographer, 'What the HELL is that?'

The radiographer, who appears to be a teenager, answers nonchalantly. 'That's your bladder, you need to empty it.'

'But I emptied it before!'

'Well, you need to empty it again.'

I've been in this hospital now for almost ten hours. I meet Simon to go for a consultation with the financial advisor for Macmillan in the hospital foyer, our precarious situation as freelance music journalists now significantly more precarious if I can't work properly in the forthcoming year. It's three weeks since I signed a deal for my very first attempt at ghostwriting a book, a memoir with Amy Winehouse's lifelong best friend, a sometime singer/songwriter-turned-farmer in Ireland, Tyler James. His mission: to reset the narrative around Amy who was never, as he put it, 'just another fuck-up who was always going to die'. I don't know, now, if I'll be able to write it; the deadline is in eight months' time, during six of which I'll be poisoned. The advisor secures us everything she can, a £365 Macmillan grant for any home essentials we might be missing (most newly diagnosed cancer patients, she smiles, opt for a new oven), which I plan to squirrel away. (A couple of months later I'll spend the lot on a new kettle, a gas/electricity bill and a vacuum cleaner. I haven't had a vacuum cleaner since the 1990s.

It's a standard cordless Sharp and it's so impressive I'll even start enthusiastically vacuuming the walls.)

Exiting the hospital in a traumatised daze, certain I have bone cancer, I'm not only wondering how I'll function generally before the official diagnosis on 23 December, but just how far this thing has taken up squatters' rights in my body. Naturally, we go to the nearest pub, mere yards away, where I'm crushed, stressed, believing I'm definitely going to die. Any casual observer, though, would believe I was more concerned about the job I now surely couldn't do, saying over and over again, 'How will I write this book?' It seemed obvious: I won't be able to write it. I'll be sick, exhausted, bedridden, for months and months and months. Won't I? Isn't that what chemo does? Isn't it The Worst? For the first time I realise I have no idea whatsoever what chemotherapy actually does to you, or even *for* you. But I still wouldn't know how bad things were, or not, for another four days. It is, as we're always told, 'the not knowing that kills you'.

We go home, drink wine, eat homemade pizza and watch a Marx Brothers movie. Only altered states, delicious food and absurdism can comfort me now. Even if, unbeknownst, the first two of those central life pleasures will soon be taken away from me altogether.

23 December 2019.

We're walking, me 'n' Simon, as rigid as a pair of ironing boards, into a consultation room adjacent to Dr Bridger's, to be met by her assistant, Dr Farah, a softly spoken, sweet-natured woman in a headscarf who is taking us through the scan results. Many documents are spread out on her table awaiting my signature, giving consent to the pouring into my body of the necessary poisons for the cell-obliterating goal ahead and therefore assigning the consequences only to myself and not the medics who are attempting to save my life.

Fair do's the NHS, the world is full of nutters.

Dr Farah: 'The cancer hasn't spread anywhere.'

'What?'

'Yes, the results are clear.'

'Really? You mean I don't have bone cancer?'

'No bone cancer, no.'

'So ... what was the "hot spot" in the scan?'

'Er ... we don't actually have the bone scan results back yet ...'

'What!?'

'... but it's probably fibroids or could be arthritis, probably nothing to worry about at all.'

'So, how do you know I don't have bone cancer?'

(Patiently): 'We'd be able to detect that from the other scans anyway.'

'Oh ... OK! So ... it's really only breast cancer I have then?'

'That's right. And I'll need you to fill in these forms ...'

Bloody hell! I'm gonny live! If all goes to plan!

Ten minutes later, after much signing and nodding and agreeing, I'm free to go, my chemotherapy start date now confirmed as 6 January 2020.

I cannot believe what I've just heard, I feel there must be some mistake. I was *convinced*. I sit bolted to my seat and the doctor waits, tolerantly, for me to leave. Simon stands up, encouraging me to *just leave*.

'Are you *sure* I don't have bone cancer?'

'You don't have bone cancer.'

'Mental!'

I skip out the door, throw my arms around Simon. 'It's going to be all right!'

We head straight back to the nearby pub, where I text all my friends and family: 'Letting you all know I've had my scan results back and they're all clear! I seriously thought I had bone cancer – it's probably fibroids, or arthritis (!?), confirmation to come – but zero indication of cancer anywhere else. Chemo starts Jan 6. Am now going to stop thinking/talking/worrying about this and get my head into Christmas. Am now in the pub with Simon and the darts is on ... everything is back to normal-ish! I only have breast cancer! This is gonny be the best Christmas EVER.'

On the bus home the feeling of elation is dizzying. I have cancer, yes, it's still officially incurable as diseases go, and the thing about cancer is it delights in coming back, but today's state-of-the-art chemical warfare can pretty much eradicate it, or keep it at bay, for years. No one can ever know if it will return, but that's for the future, the same as anyone else's future: the unknown. So I now know, as my younger self could never have known, that it's possible to have a cancer diagnosis and feel delivered of good news: this could all have been so much worse. Everything, ultimately, is perspective.

Gavin's been on my mind, who died from cancer out of nowhere. He was one of the unlucky ones and I was not. So, this Christmas, more than any other, I would be living my very own version of my favourite film of all time, *It's A Wonderful Life* (because that's the kind of sap I am).

Except, I won't be having the best Christmas ever. As a wise old saying goes: 'If you want to make God laugh, tell him your plans.'

6

WONDERFUL CHRISTMASTIME

It had been a tough twelve months for Simon. Back in 2018, one of his own best friends from boyhood had received his own devastating news: his wife was diagnosed with a life-threatening disease and this one was terminal. Simon travelled to Scotland immediately, to be whatever support he could be while tests were under way in hospital.

Less than twelve months later my diagnosis came and, in those clock-ticking days of waiting for my results, through his barely acknowledged forty-eighth birthday, he'd been inwardly planning the details of my funeral, from the location to the playlist to the sensitivities of the seating arrangements. After the 'good' news on the 23rd, on Christmas Eve, he walked up to Muswell Hill for a breather, a coffee and a think. He noticed they were showing the latest *Star Wars* movie in the Everyman, and despite loathing the previous one, decided that's what he needed for a brief respite from reality: to watch *The Rise of Skywalker*, on his own, in the afternoon, as befits a proper *Star Wars* geek.

Simon is a quietly private person. Despite a sensitive, creative nature, he is Mr Inscrutable, not given to dramatic expressions of emotion. Since all this began for us he'd never truly broken down, determined to stay strong for me. There in the cinema he was transported back to his seven-year-old self, at the pictures with his dad watching the first *Star Wars* movie, a spirited, romantic, imaginative boy who was so excited when the Death Star exploded he threw up in his seat. He thought about the boy he was then and the man he is today, about what he'd done with his life and what was being asked of him now, to deal with the difficult stuff, the grown-up stuff of life. As a pivotal, nostalgic scene unfolded, the inner dam finally burst; he sobbed openly in his seat, in the dark, alone, months of pressure expelling from his body. Things for his friend and wife were better, her response to medication was good; I wasn't about to die; he could finally look ahead to Christmas. He could do with a good blowout, no more funeral playlists pulsing at the back of his mind.

Simon is not a druggy person. He'd barely touched a drug in his life when I first met him aged thirty, had never smoked a cigarette, was an enthusiast merely of the pint of lager and the quality single-malt whisky. And, even after several of those, the most dramatic result is purple-faced giggling and a sudden creative impulse: to fashion the shape of a dancing person on the living-room floor out of discarded clothes, coasters, eye masks, empty cans and artificial flowers as soon as I've gone to bed, to 'surprise' me in the morning. Some of my friends, however, remain marijuana devotees and, in the last decade, for Simon's birthday, have gifted him a small handful of weed, which he's found rather pleasant for a special occasion. Nowadays an occasional cigar smoker, he simply smokes the weed with some festive baccy as an experiment in sonic enhancement, conjuring an even greater appreciation of his Jimi Hendrix albums on vinyl and, er, that's about it.

This year he decides the special occasion is Christmas Day, the best Christmas ever, seeing as I'm not about to die. This year, though, for shady supply-chain reasons, he's not been given flaky, fragrant weed, but cannabis resin, the small, black block you heat with a lighter and crumble like an Oxo cube. He loathes resin, after living with students in the early nineties who smoked it constantly; even the smell makes him queasy. A plan B emerges: after *Star Wars* he buys brownie mix from Sainsbury's and, on Christmas Day, after our delicious meal, bakes all the resin into a space cake, with no clue about quantity, and eats it. All of it.

Simultaneously, the TV goes down. We lose the signal, a problem seemingly with the communal block arial. So instead of watching the Queen's Christmas message like the rest of the country, we're ploughing through a *Laurel and Hardy* boxset, followed by a Christmas episode of *Frasier*. Not that Simon takes any of this in because, half an hour after munching through his gritty Christmas bake, he loses his mind. He's hallucinating rainbow streaks of colour, his heart speeding up with panic-attack palpitations, the pale blue irises of his wide-open eyes disappearing under the top lid, so his eye sockets are now a hundred per cent milky white. I'm screaming, 'Wake up! Drink some water! Come back!', convinced it is now *he* who is about to die. I poke him constantly to make sure he stays awake, his eyeless head lolling onto the back of the sofa, hand him litres of water and wait for this madness to subside. His heart, eventually, slows down, his eyes return to his head. Mortified, shaken and exhausted, he heads off early to bed.

We both wake up on Boxing Day. That'll do for a start. He's still traumatised, vows he'll never touch the stuff again, and I know he never will. I'm far more gutted than annoyed: I've understood, for ever, this impulse to escape. Reality is often hard. Sometimes, you just need your head to be somewhere else, 'out of it' indeed, and all he wanted was a few hours of alternative reality, full of music and jokes and colours. Instead? A cardiac event, hallucination panic and eyeless catatonia. Today, already not the best Boxing Day ever, I've promised I'll visit a neighbour who's on her own and struggling, currently bedbound in the middle of gruelling chemotherapy for womb cancer.

Two hours later I stagger back through our front door in a state of advanced anxiety, having listened to a verbal landslide of chemo side-effect horrors: nerve damage causing inability to feel anything from the knees down, constant nausea, no taste, diarrhoea and constipation 'at exactly the same time', complete loss of hair, trembling hands due to steroids. Yet she has to somehow drive herself to hospital every single day, for three weeks, to undergo radiotherapy. I'm very thankful, as New Year's Eve approaches, I'm still able to have a festive drink, because from 2 January onwards I'll be giving up booze completely, for six months, until chemotherapy is over. Happy New Year!

Chemo Suite Introduction Day, 2 January.

Nadia is the gentlest woman on Earth, a specialist cancer nurse from Slovakia who guides me over to a reclining bed-chair where I'll sit, legs stretched outwards, while I'm hooked up to various intravenous drips. The purpose of today is to prepare me for 'the process' to come and everything here is alien. There's the treatment machine plugged into the wall: a digital chemotherapy pump, like a nineties' Amstrad computer, fitted onto a drip stand on castors which always reminds me of Tom Hanks dying in *Philadelphia*. The treatment process, as well as chemo, will regularly include intravenous antibody infusions, and many tube-clearing saline flushes in between, meaning some weeks treatment will take a full eight hours. Nadia swishes the regulation blue hospital curtain around us for privacy and forensically details all the possible chemo side effects (around fifty of them, terrifyingly), including signs of a potentially fatal blood clot which must entail the immediate ringing of an ambulance. She mentions the other nurses who'll look after me, one of whom is called Prince.

'Prince?' I blurt out loud. 'There's a Prince?'

The blue curtain twitches and a friendly, handsome face peers through. 'I'm Prince.'

'Delighted to meet you!'

'See you again soon …'

Back home, derealisation is giving way to a painfully sharp focus and I dread what lies ahead. Despite the constant presence today of cancer diagnoses, whether in our families, friends or in public figures, despite the one-in-two-of-us statistics, despite the leaflet-dispensing nurses and the hours of obsessional googling – I'm aware I *still* don't fully understand what 'chemotherapy' specifically means, even five weeks post-diagnosis. You only ever hear that it's 'gruelling'. With no descriptive details. Perhaps no one wants to hear them. Perhaps it's too distressing. Perhaps no one wants to appear ungrateful, or not 'strong' or not 'brave'. Perhaps no one loves a whinger. But I *do* want to know.

We all know the gist: you'll be 'tired', possibly even bedridden, have a few mouth ulcers, your hair will fall out, maybe some *unusual* bathroom activity. But how bad can it be? Maybe it's not that bad? Or maybe it'll be worse than I ever could have imagined? The brain churns on.

I'm going to be properly ill now. Isn't that what always happens? Will I be any good at being this ill? What kind of ill will it be? How ill can *you be and still function? What if I really can't work? I've got no insurance; I can't afford to not work. If I lose the flat I'm finished. Which means so is Simon. Oh God, poor Simon, he'll become my carer and he's only in his forties! And I'm really* really *sorry about that.*

Puffs on my beloved vape become ever more urgent, the chemical release and relief bringing with it a pummelling thud of regret. I wonder why it was I started smoking in the first place and Ali's face comes beaming, as ever, into view.

7

REGRETS (AND FAGS)
I'VE HAD A FEW

We weren't just uncool; we were laughably uncool. As thirteen-year-olds starting secondary school we'd made a 'pact': we wouldn't succumb to what we somehow thought were 'tarty' black tights and instead would stick with our sappy, white, primary-school socks. We strode into first year not only in our weedy socks but wielding shiny, girly-swot *briefcases*. We might as well have painted late-seventies' mod revival targets on our backs. The skinhead tough girls duly took aim, especially at me, a sickly blonde with lumpy-kneed, stringy legs. They shouldered me, poking my back, pointing at the briefcase and cackling like cockatoos.

Soon me 'n' Ali turned fourteen and, like all fourteen-year-olds, wished to grow up, toughen up and at least *attempt* to be cool. So we decided: let's start smoking!

We both worked weekends and occasional weekday nights behind the counter of the café in Bell's Sports Centre, the spaceship on the North Inch, for 50p an hour. Too young to buy cigarettes, we stole ten Regal out of the in-shop drawer, darted into the park post-work and loitered by a towering cedar tree. Placing snouts on eager lips, Ali sparked a lighter and we both enthusiastically inhaled. And coughed and coughed like emphysemic 1970s beagles. Disgusting, we thought. But we were determined, we persevered. Eventually, I liked the rush, the tingle on the surface of the scalp.

Soon we were unstoppable, i.e. addicted. The ice-cream van parked outside the school sold single cigarettes, alongside the Quavers and Marathon bars we bought with our daily dinner money. I'd buy what was known as 'a single' and join the many pals who were already smokers, loitering on the edge of the playground. I stole single fags from my mum's permanent packets of Benson & Hedges and a metamorphosis was on its way. It would've happened anyway: wearing the 'tarty' black tights, smoking every day, the briefcase ditched for a light-blue canvas satchel meticulously biroed with the logos of the bands I was now obsessed with: The Who, The Jam, The Specials, Madness, The Police.

Most crucially of all, with extra cash from my parents for my fifteenth birthday, I had my weedy long hair cut off into a post-punk elfin crop, dyed peroxide blonde. Their cash contribution was no doubt a source of regret: from this day on, to my horrified mum, I was 'a monster from outer space'. The tough girls faded away and my life was changed for ever.

Soon, me 'n' Ali would smoke the full spectrum of cigarettes, from long, cigarillo-style More cigarettes, to Consulate menthols, to Regal King Size. Ali stole singles from her dad's packets of Player's No. 6; he noticed and switched to pungently macho Woodbine attempting to put her off. She had a go on his pipe instead. From '79 onwards, I would be a smoker of something, on and off – cigarettes, roll-ups, through the evolution of vapes – for the next forty-two years. That's a lot of opportunity for a human cell, just one, to mutate and multiply and, eventually, even decades later, kill me.

I'd tried to give up several times: acupuncture, twice, jolting on a consultation day bed as pins were lodged in ears. It worked!

For three months, each time. Back in '97 I had my first vape, a rudimentary, first-generation plastic pipe with a mouthpiece, which looked like a cross between a kazoo and a tampon, a not yet widely known gizmo which made former Led Zeppelin compadres Robert 'Percy' Plant and Jimmy 'the air of a man who's done many bad things' Page, snort in disbelief during an interview at 'an *NME* journalist sucking on a piece of plastic!?'

In the 2000s I tried hypnotherapy above a health-food store, encouraged to envisage indoor bonfires of lit cigarettes and acrid smoke, against pine forests of oxygenised freshness. I walked out with a clanging headache, which lasted three days, alleviated only when I started smoking again. Yours, madam, for £125. I gave up three times when pregnant, for as long as the pregnancies lasted, before three miscarriages between five weeks and three months. I gave up once for a whole year and have no idea how it was possible to start again.

And now, here in my fifties, I'm as addicted to the fruity nicotine temptations of the contemporary vaporiser as I have been to anything else. I know I know better than this. I watched my mum smoke herself to death, a chain-smoker for decades who spent the last few years of her life with an oxygen nebuliser at home which she'd breathe through, on and off, in between the Benson & Hedges, until chronic obstructive pulmonary disease (COPD) brutally finished her off. I knew it couldn't go on. And yet, here, in January 2020, in the middle of a traumatising life event, giving the vape up any time soon is unthinkable.

What's bothering me much more, in fact, is how I'll get through eight hours in a chemotherapy chair without it.

8

NEW YEAR, NEW YOU
(NOT A GOOD LOOK)

I'm on the bus again with Simon, this time without his knee being gripped as if by a pair of pliers. We're off to my first chemotherapy session and while not exactly looking forward to this in the way you would, say, a day trip to Chessington World of Adventures, I am up for it.

Let the science commence! Let the pollution begin! Let's get on with it so I can get back to normal as sharpish as possible and all this, one day, will seem an outrageously vivid fever dream and I'm going to live to be 109 after all. Hopefully. If I stay lucky. Maybe?

Inside the clinic, with my legs stretched along the reclining seat, a bag of saline is hooked on the top of a pole on castors, a thin cannula tube snaking down to the needle attached to the back of my hand. The nurse overseeing my first chemo session will be Bimpe, originally from Nigeria, the chemo unit's head nurse.

First, though, before the poisoning can begin, my hair is gently water sprayed by a young nurse, Mel, then combed through with conditioner, in preparation for the rigours of the cold cap. I've never seen one before; it's like an ice-hockey helmet, streamlined and hard on the outside, with an inner lining of gel, attached via bendy hose to a small, refrigerated machine that pumps in coolant to freeze the hair follicles and what feels like my entire brain. Mel wedges the cap tight to my skull, flips the 'on' switch and waves of crinkling sounds flow around my head, a freezing process I can clearly hear, instantaneous ice contracting all the way around the scalp. It's agonising, as if I've bolted down five litres of ice cream in one, a biting, constant 'burn' turning my brain into a Slush Puppie.

Simon sits by the bed, trying to distract me with a barrage of difficult, memory-jogging questions, which works, but this is *pain*. After twenty minutes I'm ready to abandon the cap – it's only hair, it'll grow back again – when the breakthrough happens, a numbness, a sudden sensation of tolerance; *I can handle this*. The cap stays on for the full three hours.

I'm half an hour into brain freeze when Bimpe sits by me with a bag of neon crimson poison, a liquid so toxic she must inject it manually through a syringe into the cannula wearing surgical gloves – it's too risky a substance to be dangled overhead on the pole. She tells me, warmly and matter-of-factly, that the next six months 'will be a bit of a slog'. She adds, with a hoot of laughter, 'but in my country they leave you to die in the street!'

I'm despatched homewards with several packets of pills (to stave off approaching side effects): steroids, anti-sickness pills, anti-diarrhoea pills. (This week, I'll buy a daily pill organiser from Superdrug and feel like I'm living in a care home already, a Perspex box which now permanently resides below the kitchen calendar featuring scenes of bonnie Scotland. Perhaps I *am* living in a care home already.)

Back home I feel so normal I wonder if anything has actually *gone in*. I'm disorientated, light-headed, but nothing too unusual. And then, around 7 p.m., my heart rate suddenly accelerates. Terrifyingly. I can feel the full shape of my heart pounding in my chest, like it's coming loose, wobbling, while my teeth begin uncontrollably chattering, as if I'm horrifyingly cold, in hypothermic shock. But it's nothing to do with temperature, it's neurological bedlam, like coming up on a dodgy E back in the 1990s.

Don't take me back there!

Staggering into the bedroom, hands quivering, I sit down on the bed, bend forward and try to deep breathe, deep breathe, to make this thing stop, convinced there'll be an imminent cardiac arrest. It lasts a *full forty minutes*. Eventually the wave ebbs away, a normal heart rate returns, leaving me exhausted, traumatised. I slip into bed and endure a night of terror-filled non-sleep, certain my heart will suddenly give up.

The next morning I must return to hospital for a pelvic scan to determine the nature of the bone scan 'hot spot' (in the weeks to come, benign fibroids will thankfully be confirmed). Detouring into the chemo ward, Bimpe reassures me: my Cardiac Event was normal, it could be the steroids, could be the chemo itself, my body adjusting to the shock of alien toxins. It won't be as bad from now on.

The first full day passes. The weirdest thing is that I *don't* feel weird, I feel weirdly normal. That evening, though, while having a pasta tea, a forkful of food somehow refuses to slip down my throat, it just sits at the back of the tongue, so I have to swallow and swallow and swallow, forcing it down. My voice, too, is sounding slightly... husky.

It's week one of the six-month no alcohol rule I've imposed on myself: general chemo attacks your liver because it attacks *everything*, every single cell in your body, both healthy and cancerous (nuking, hopefully, all the rogue ones along the way) and I'm going to need that liver when this is all over – when I'm back in a cosy pub, pint of delicious Strongbow aloft. I'm playing the long game.

News arrives that a fellow journalist has died of breast cancer,

America's Elizabeth Wurtzel, author of the nineties' landmark memoir *Prozac Nation*. As so often happens when your peers die, I immediately compare my age to hers. She is two years younger than I am. This is alarming, so now I'm alarming myself even further, googling other instances of writers dying of recurring breast cancer. There are many. American *Interview* magazine legend Ingrid Sischy in 2015, thirteen years older than I am. Deborah Orr in 2019, three years older than I am. I'm now tormented by the thought of recurrence, paralysed by The Fear.

It will come back, I know it will, I'm not lucky like that, I just know I'm not.

Days pass and I'm still feeling weirdly normal. The skin on my face is so clear I look like I've been on a week-long detox retreat in the Austrian Alps, which may be the result of five days off the booze.

I'm still wondering when I'll succumb to The Hole when a hospital pharmacist rings, also wondering if I've experienced 'the dip' yet. She advises it might happen when I stop taking steroids, the last of which I've just taken. I'm feeling, if anything, euphoric, going for walks around Alexandra Park, which lies directly across from our flat, currently bathed in clear-skied January sunshine. For years now my heroes have evolved from musical to existential, from artistic to holistic, my greatest inspiration today the nature punk Chris Packham, who speaks more eloquently than even David Attenborough Himself on the healing power of nature.

More days pass and I'm becoming woozily spaced out, as if on strong painkillers, and feel much hungrier than usual. We have a Chinese takeaway, the spices from which I can feel penetrating my scalp, the flavours a sensory overload of deliciousness, making me feel euphoric again, as you would with a runner's high. Simultaneously, most days now, I'm passing out by 8.30 p.m., head nod-nod-nodding while watching TV, which I fight until 10.30 p.m. I then wake up at 3.15 a.m., my unusually clear skin now replaced by inflamed red patches dotted around my face. From now on I keep waking up at 2, 3, 4 a.m., while constipation impudently turns up.

Fourteen days after the first poisoning I awake at a frankly log-slept 5 a.m. and feel like someone has traced a blowtorch around the inside of my mouth, and throat, voice plummeting towards a baritone 'Barry White'. My mouth is disintegrating, large white patches of mouth ulcer breaking out inside the cheeks, along the tongue, inside the lips. Eating is now excruciating. I'm frighteningly cold, deep frozen to the bone, teeth clattering together, upper body trembling. I simply put up with it. This must be the expected 'dip'.

Ali rings to see how I'm doing and I make light of it: the mouth is bad but I'll just eat ice cream! Even though I'm freezing already. She's alarmed but reassured. I've an appointment soon with the doc. Just as well: I'm now having problems swallowing anything, my whole tongue feels tender and sore. I can't brush my teeth any more, it's torturous, so use a salt gargle, take paracetamol and hope it fades away. It doesn't. It gets worse, as if a swarm of wasps has flown into my mouth, performed a series of pirouetting sting manoeuvres and flown out again. My inner goth knows: this isn't turning out well.

Monday 20 January 2020, 1 p.m.

The day of my first regular post-chemo review appointment with Dr Bridger is finally here. I'm so relieved: *I really need to see The Doctor*. Arriving at the clinic reception with Simon I'm told there's no appointment in the system. It's too early for my first chemo review. I'd feel like John McEnroe in 1982 if I didn't feel so feeble: *you cannot be serious!* Tears stab at my eyes. The receptionist tells me he will somehow make this appointment happen, come back in two hours. We head to the canteen; I'm hungry and yet not hungry. It's 1 p.m. and I should be. I decide to attempt a decaf latte after it's cooled down; Simon asks what I'd like to eat. I don't know. I'm frightened to eat, it's so painful. Simon is exasperated, he knows I need to eat properly and harangues me, *choose something.* I choose a banana. Seated at a canteen table, a small bite of banana burns like a piece of coal newly tonged from an open fire.

Tears flow from a crushing sense of helplessness, of feeling I just can't cope, of not knowing what to do. I need medication, I'm scared, I'm hopeless, I'm useless. I'm wearing a shirt, a jumper, a winter coat and a scarf and I can't stop shivering, now violently shaking with cold. Hospitals are never cold. By 3 p.m., back in the clinic, the receptionist has worked his magic: Dr Bridger will see you now. Seated before her once more, she asks questions: how have you been? OK until the last forty-eight hours. She shines a light inside my ulcerated mouth, peers down my blowtorched throat, takes my temperature. 37.3. Nothing too ominous.

Nonetheless she tells me, 'I think you need to go to ambulatory care,' and I've no idea what that means. 'I'm asking for blood tests, to check for sepsis.'

Sepsis? Whoever said anything about sepsis!? I know about sepsis, it can kill you, pretty much instantly, if you go into septic shock.

'I could send you home and say take paracetamol,' she adds, 'but I think you'd be back here in an hour, in an ambulance.'

What!?!?

In ambulatory care, an emergency wing of the hospital less hectic than A&E, nurses take blood samples, five large tubes of blood – 'that's nearly an armful!' as Tony Hancock once said – then send for immediate diagnosis. My temperature is rapidly ascending, 38.9, I'm still shivering, now hooked up to an antibiotic drip. The diagnosis arrives: I have something called 'neutropenic sepsis'. My neutrophil count is 0.1, where the normal range is between 2.0 and 7.5. Less than 0.5 is officially defined as 'severely neutropenic'. All of which means my white blood cells have crashed to zero and my immune system is on the floor, at its lowest point in the chemo cycle, leaving me with nothing to fight any infection. Not that I knew that until I googled it:

How serious is neutropenic sepsis?

Neutropenic sepsis is a potentially fatal complication of anticancer treatment (particularly chemotherapy). Mortality rates ranging between 2 per cent and 21 per cent have been reported in adults.

Twenty-one per cent. *One in five.* That sounds a *certainty* to me. If the receptionist hadn't made sure I saw the doctor, I might have just gone home, feeling ill and weepy, taken paracetamol, gone to bed wearing three jumpers, woollen leggings and thermal socks and been dead by the middle of the night. Instead, I'm placed on a hospital trolley, drip still attached, awaiting an empty bed in a side room. My inner goth was both right and wrong. In some important ways, I seem to be getting luckier and luckier. Though I won't feel it over the coming days, when I'm incarcerated in hospital, which makes me understand more clearly the information signs you see in hospital toilets, the ones which plead, 'When can I go home?'

9

THE NEEDLE AND THE DAMAGE DONE

Being suddenly told you're being taken into hospital for an indeterminate time is a moment of surreal bewilderment. Your mind pads around in confusion fretting about clean underwear, mobile-phone chargers, even pyjamas. As if a hospital won't provide you with the regulation, diamond-motif gown and make you sit in bed with your jumper on.

I'm in a side room all to myself, feeling relieved at my supposed good fortune of privacy until I realise my own naivety: I've been quarantined – if any infection reaches me, having zero immune system, I am doomed. For this reason, in January 2020, even though Covid is still a faraway whisper, all the nurses, doctors and visitors must wear masks, the likes of which I've only ever seen on TV or on the faces of Japanese tourists taking photos of Buckingham Palace guards in comedy bearskin hats.

Whenever anyone comes in, mostly nurses wheeling the 'obs' machine (two-to-four hourly observations of blood pressure, oxygen level and temperature), I feel like E.T., when the scientists trap him in the antiseptic tent surrounded by anonymous humans wearing full PPE. Until now, I've never heard the term personal protective equipment, or seen it in reality; masks, gloves and cling-filmy blue aprons, all of which are dumped in a bin (surely a recycling bin) the moment they wheel back out the door. My temperature is 38.9 while my body still quakes with chills but I'm much relieved to be 'in the right place'. Sadly, and I don't have the heart to complain, the light in the loo doesn't work.

Hooked up to drip bags of industrial antibiotics, delivered via yet another cannula, I'm hypnotised by the constant, rhythmic sound of the digital feeding machine – pshsht! pshsht! pshsht! – which gives way, when the drip bags are empty, to an incessant *beep-beep-beep*, an aggravating alarm it takes the nurses up to an hour to respond to, which means, while I'm waiting, I've gone *completely mad*.

Ali rings, learns of the sepsis and breaks down in highly uncharacteristic tears. 'I knew I should've said something,' she blurts, 'but I didn't want to scare you. I knew this could happen but not this soon. I should've told you to get to the hospital right away!'

She's so upset I'm now upset.

'Are you trying to tell me the doctor saved my life?'

'Sylv, I think she did. But a doctor would never say that.'

An NHS doctor has saved my life already, then, *and* the receptionist before her. For them? Just one more day at the office.

For five days and five nights I'm imprisoned, moved out of the 'acute' ward to a different side room on day two, where at least the light in the toilet works. This length of hospital stay is an adult lifetime first. Every day, every hour, is an education.

You never sleep. For a start, those regular obs don't let up through the night, a nurse wheeling the machine into your room, light clicked on, every two/three hours until daybreak when, in my case, a blood test is taken which would certainly wake anyone up if they weren't gungy-eyed awake already. My side room is off the respiratory ward and all night long, while lying awake, I hear the rasping, phlegmy and guttural hacking of lungs which no longer work. It's stiflingly hot, permanently. One night, I feel around in the dark for my phone on the bedside table to check the time. No phone. I panic, sit up, switch on the light. No phone anywhere. I look in every drawer, in the loo, behind the bed, in the bed, then strip the bed, hoist up the mattress. Still no phone. Convinced one of the nurses has taken it by accident, I pad out to reception to ask everyone to check, to be told I must've forgotten to bring my phone. One hour later a nurse walks in with it in her hand: she did take it by accident, hers is identical. I'm now plugged back into the life-support machine, my only connection to everyone and everything in the outside world: all the humans I'm desperate to communicate with, all the news I need to know, all the googling of information I suddenly must have and the vital role, in my current situation, of infinite distraction. We know we lived without them, for millennia. But *how?* Never let anyone tell you we're not addicted to our phones, their properties as powerful and insidious as heroin.

I learn how painful blood tests and cannulas can be. My veins are non-existent in the crook of my arm, better in the back of the hand, the most painful site apparently. One morning at 6 a.m. two nurses try four times between them to extract blood, the murderously stingy jabs refusing to yield a drop. Blood test results are my only hope of a passport home so if they can't take blood I'll be staying here until I'm dead. Eventually, the requisite rivers come, the back of my hand soon as alien to me as a ninety-five-year-old stranger's, a huge blue/purple blob with seeping tendrils where distinct veins used to be, the result not only of all that stabbing but, I'm told, 'very strong antibiotics'. Soon, my hand stops giving *any* blood, the veins on strike, so more jabbing in the arm crook ensues, resulting in cotton wool pads taped all over the back of the hand and inner arm. Nurses tell me how reasonable I'm being, how men are notoriously so much worse with needles than women, very quick to complain about pain, to declare themselves 'needle phobic', with much squirming and yelping and general dramatics, *the saps*.

Doctors, I now know, turn up unexpectedly and do unexpected things. One morning I'm asked by a nurse if my bowels 'have moved today?' They have, slightly, which caused me serious pain, which I feel obliged to blab about. A young female doctor and her male student doctor then stride through the door announcing the requirement of 'a rectal examination'. Blue rubber gloves are snapped on as she asks me to lie on my side, nightie up, knickers off, lift the outer knee to my chin. From the corner of my eye I see cool blue gel administered to gloved middle finger and – aaaiiiieeeee! – a sharp, shooting pain blazes from the icy finger, which quickly (mercifully) retracts. 'No fissures' is the official diagnosis although she's detected 'one haemorrhoid'. A conversation ensues between myself and the young student doctor about the nature of the pain in the anus of his middle-aged female patient, while I inwardly think, Seriously, young man, are you *sure* you want to be a doctor?

I'd wondered, before I was incarcerated, if hospital food could possibly be as bad as we're always told. Each morning you're given an A4 piece of paper with the day's menu to select from, both 'Lunch' and what they rather middle-classily call 'Supper' to be chosen at the same time. One day I have an 'appetiser' of mushroom soup, which arrives in a beige plastic disposable cup, the ones you got from a vending machine in the 1970s. A now-cold baked potato comes in tinfoil straight from the microwave, with one plastic tub of tuna mayonnaise, three golden-foil-wrapped portions of butter, two sachets of salad cream and one plastic tub of side salad (sliced tomato, bit of lettuce, sweetcorn). All of it tastes of absolutely nothing. Other seventies' delights include: chicken stuffing sandwich on white, pear halves in juice, with custard, and a hot chocolate which also arrives in the beige cup from the vending machine in 1976. In my condition, to add injury to insult (with genuine apologies to the NHS budget which I fully understand does not prioritise Michelin-star cuisine), every mouthful of this dreadful fare can only be tolerated after two paracetamols and a large swill of Difflam mouthwash, my pain-relief saviour, which numbs the mouth; so even if this *was* Michelin-star cuisine it would taste of wasp stings and antiseptic floor cleaner anyway. To distract from the daily starvation, I'm watching my favourite sport, snooker, on my laptop, which Simon has heroically brought in, after first sending texts detailing the games I've missed so far.

'Judd Trump just been beaten by a fifty-four-year-old I've never heard of!' he pings. 'The name's Bond. Nigel Bond. John Parrot said he "played the living daylights out of him" etc. Licensed to pot. The man with the golden cue. I can hear it all now!'

One day I'm sent for a chest X-ray, a cheery cockney hospital porter turning up in the room with a wheelchair, which protocol insists I sit in, even though I can walk, 'because some people have been known to faint'. Wheeling towards the X-ray department I see patients grappling with crutches, while one beardy man, maybe fifty, lies on a hospital trolley, his face spectrally pale and emotionally blank, not far it seems to me from death. I now know how it feels to be in an episode of *24 Hours in A&E*. After the X-ray, bare breasts pressed up against a metal plate, I'm not yet dressed when the porter returns. 'Oh sorry, I'll wait!' To speed things up I simply put my jumper on, stuffing my bra inside. Wheeled back inside my room, I stand up and the black bra shoots out from under the jumper, skidding into the middle of the floor. Hysteria ensues. The porter waves me goodbye with the chipper parting message, 'You gotta laugh ain't yer!?'

You do, especially when you also must endure the dismal 'light' that permeates all hospitals. Light is important. Without it, the Earth would die and so would we, within months, were we to live within these walls full time. Overhead, grey squares are consecutively lit a watery urine-yellow, in a largely windowless world. My room, thankfully, has thin slats of window, but it's winter, and grey, with barely one dusty beam of natural light penetrating the gloom. It feels like living in a bleary-eyed 3 a.m. netherworld. The excellent KLF song '3 a.m. Eternal', I'm now convinced, is a song about staying in hospital.

How the staff cope with this aspect of hospital life alone is heroic, a staff that come from all over the world. How could the NHS function, I wonder many times, without immigration? Many of the nurses (and porters and cleaners) have come to the UK from every corner of the planet to work for the NHS specifically: Greece, Spain, Ireland, Japan, Indonesia, many countries of eastern Europe, all corners of Africa. Many are the descendants of the Windrush generation. Some are quiet and stoic, some boisterous and quick with the quips, like a nurse I inwardly call Comedy Tito, from Jamaica, who knocks every time he's about to come in. 'Don't mind me!' he always announces, grinning, followed by, 'As they say in Jamaica, it's gonna be *aaaahl-right*.' You succumb, quickly, to Stockholm syndrome, feeling not only physically but emotionally dependent on these people, your captors and tormentors.

Humiliation continues to be a way of life. I learn how to steer the treatment pole across the floor to the toilet, often on wayward, twirling castors, the digital pump now unplugged from the wall and sending out its alarm, *beep-beep-beep*. It's the same piercing alarm sound as the empty drip-bag alert, which can only be switched off by a nurse, and only then can I be detached from the pole and untethered from the cannula tube.

I'm still waiting for a nurse to release me one morning when I'm having my Weetabix and sliced banana. Suddenly, I feel the unmistakable internal shift of bowel looseness. Emptiness is imminent. *Oh no.* Rapidly unplugging the machine, hastily draping the plug and cable over the hook at the top of the pole, I'm shuffling at speed towards the loo, squeezing everything in, shuffle-shuffle-shuffle, attempting to haul down knickers and pyjama bottoms with one hand at the requisite accident-avoiding angle, only to *not* make it to the pan on time.

With no time to put the light on, it's all out there in the semi-darkness, inside my knickers, pyjama bottoms, on the grey-tiled toilet floor. Switching the light on, I take the offending clothes off, clean myself and the floor with toilet paper, when the phone begins to ring and ring, three separate times. It's Simon, panicking, telling me he's just been sent, somehow, an accidental message from me, consisting of nothing but the *beep–beep–beep* of the digital machine, which sounded to him like a heart monitor flatlining. He's convinced it was my dying message from an operating table.

'I was freaking out!' he's shouting, 'I thought you were dying!' while I'm standing naked from the waist down wondering what the hell happened to life as I knew it. Knickers and pyjama bottoms are washed in the sink with shower gel, wrung out and hung limply over the visitors' chair. Horrified, this is the nearest I've ever been to the Spud scene in *Trainspotting*, where soiled sheets accidentally unfurl over an unsuspecting family at the breakfast table. They never tell you *this* is part of 'the process'. At least, I think gratefully, it didn't happen in the room where the bathroom was in permanent darkness.

A nurse finally arrives to release me from the machine and I have to tell her what's happened, asking for the regulation hospital gown until my pyjama bottoms dry. Naturally, she's unperturbed. 'Don't worry ma'am,' she says, breezily. These people have seen it all. And it's still only 8.20 a.m. It's astonishing, I think, what you come to accept in life as your new reality. When you've no choice. When you can't fight something, whatever it is, and you just have to, in the grand Gallagher brothers tradition, roll with it.

Eventually, my neutrophil count is high enough to allow me home and I'm officially discharged, more desperate to get home than ever before in my life. I'm given self-administering injections to help generate white blood cells so I won't succumb to sepsis again – and advised to stay away, for a few days, from germy public places. My next chemotherapy, meanwhile, has been postponed a week, the original date of the following week too early for further poisoning.

Walking out of the side-room door and through the open-plan central office is surreal, the nurses and doctors all bustling, busy, heads down, things to do, patients to see and you suddenly don't exist, because they're not looking after you any more. You're nothing to them – why should you be? You're fixed – you're now a space where a full bed once was. It feels unexpectedly emotional, like saying goodbye to the world's worst hotel rooms, which have saved your life. Inside the lift, I stay pinned to the back wall with my mask on, the other three occupants potentially infectious killers. Padding down the corridors towards the exit I see bolstering quotes on walls.

'I have loved the stars too fondly to be fearful of the night' – Galileo.

Back home – glorious home! – I'm fiddling inside my wallet when I find a card I was given by Nadia on Chemo Introduction Day. It has a specific name, it's a chemotherapy alert card, displaying your details: name, hospital number, NHS number, consultant's name, the phone numbers for the chemo ward. Only now do I look at the back of the card, which I've had for nearly a month:

Important information for A&E staff and Primary Care. This patient is at risk of having neutropenic sepsis, which is a MEDICAL EMERGENCY. Refer to your local acute trust neutropenic sepsis policy immediately. DO NOT DELAY IN GIVING ANTIBOTICS. (Must be given in less than one hour of presentation.)

I blink, startled, and think, not for the first time in my life, *yooo styooopid bastid.* First rule of Cancer Club: always read any printed information you're ever given by anyone in the NHS, very carefully, at least twice.

Languishing in my coat pocket, meanwhile, is my beloved fruity vape, which I have not puffed for five days and nights, not once. I didn't even think about it because I couldn't use it. In my condition, with a mouthful of ulcerated sores, I wasn't about to swirl toxic, foggy chemicals into the open wounds of my blowtorched mucus membrane. Miraculously, I have zero nicotine cravings and I know: this is it, *finally*, a real chance to be rid of this addiction for ever. But can I just … give it up? I can. I throw the vape in a drawer and forget about it. For the first time since my teenage years, I don't think about smoking any more. I think, instead, I'll never smoke anything ever again. No longer being addicted to nicotine is the greatest unexpected positive of the longest hospital stay of my adult life. Which makes me think, for the first time in decades, of my *first* lengthy hospital stay.

The first time the NHS saved my life.

10

BORN TO BE ALIVE

Jackknifed upside down over the bottom edge of the hospital bed, I'm having my back thwack-thwack-thwacked by the kindly, firm-handed, and unforgettably named Nurse Irons, her task being to dislodge the meddlesome mucus currently clogging up my diseased lungs.

I'm six years old, it's 1971 and I have double pneumonia, which means potentially fatal disease in both lungs. I've been in Perth Royal Infirmary for weeks and almost died twice, not only from pneumonia but following a massive dose of supposedly life-saving penicillin, which it turns out I'm allergic to, skyrocketing my temperature to 104°F. Any higher and, coupled with the infection, brain damage potentially loomed.

Dad took me home, wrapped up in his hefty car coat, and carried me in his arms into the house. 'Who's this then?' he beamed to ten-year-old Jackie, who hadn't seen her wee sister for weeks, now flying towards us, arms outstretched. A doc came round for a check-up, saw a stringy-legged weakling and had some advice for my supposedly clue-free parents (one of whom was a nurse): 'She needs to build up her immune system. Put her in the garden and let her eat dirt!'

Not being too fond of the wormy soil was possibly one reason

I remained a stringy-legged weakling right up until adolescence, the years between sporadically spent in bed under a bobbly, pea-green candlewick bedspread, felled by some flu or infection, Mum's glass thermometer forever dangling out of my mouth. I never complained, this was just how things always seemed to be. One day, under the bedspread, I heard Dad say to Mum, 'I've never known a bairn that can take it like it.' And I was bairn number five. Maybe I was born with extra patience. Maybe it was my DNA: Dad had been a prisoner of war in the Second World War, surviving three and a half near-fatal years at the hands of the notoriously brutal Japanese army. Maybe it was the inner goth already crystallising in my soul, someone who's always known, any second now, every one of us could be *doomed*.

While the double-pneumonia episode was the first time the NHS saved my life, since then, if they haven't necessarily had to save it, they've done everything in their considerable power to mend the bits that have (often hideously) broken down.

As a pre-adolescent I had gruesome boils regularly sprout all over my knees, and in my twenties had similar lumps erupt around the outer edges of my breasts, which often leaked with yellow pus (don't fancy yours much, etc.). No condition was ever identified, only industrial antibiotics prescribed, which fixed it, leaving scars to this day.

Aged nineteen, now sharing my first flat in Perth with Jill and Ev, I woke up one morning with a face like a *Doctor Who* monster: angry pustular eruptions all over the cheeks, forehead and jaw, a spray of hard, white spots and blisters, eyelids fully swollen, clamping my eyes almost shut. The horrified girls alerted my parents who drove me straight to Perth Royal Infirmary A&E. From here, I was sent to Ninewells hospital, Dundee, which housed a specialist dermatology unit. From tests they surmised an allergy to the sun, shielding me behind a screen in the dermatology ward from the daylight rippling through the windows (the inner goth must've been *very* pleased). Ali visited and we could barely hear each other through the screen. No diagnosis, again, was ever reached, merely 'some kind of allergy', fixed again via antibiotics. The process of healing took weeks and eventually Ali persuaded me out in public, to a pub where no one knew us, the Clachan, where I sat indoors wearing ludicrously large shades, trying not to scare the public with my poisonous, gargoyle's face. A song came spangling out of the jukebox, a huge hit that year: Lloyd Cole And The Commotions' 'Perfect Skin'. Ali, being Ali, took no end of pleasure in roaring the song straight into my ear: 'She's got … purrfect skiiin!' One open-topped Vesuvian crater, filled with permanently oozing pus, refused to close and heal, leaving an open hole in the lower side of my face for eighteen months (*still* don't fancy yours much), which was finally stitched up when I reached London, aged twenty, at St Thomas' Hospital. A botched surgery, this left the lower right cheek badly puckered to this day.

Over the smoking years, the NHS fixed persistent bronchitis, which, had I carried on smoking, would've led to so many antibiotics throughout the decades I'd now surely have total, and fatal, immunity.

In my mid-twenties I awoke one morning to a fiery pulsing around the vaginal area; reaching down my fingers recoiled from the extensive bulge they were suddenly fondling, an egg-sized alien object living inside the labial skin. Shrieking, terrorised, I somehow didn't go to A&E, but my local GP instead, hobbling all the way as if on horseback, begging to be seen immediately. The doc, after a second's glance, and announcing the words 'labial cyst', had me ambulanced off to A&E where I was saturated with morphine, placed on a trolley and wheeled in for emergency surgery. Off my rocker on the world's best drugs I yelped, 'I love you all!' to every approaching staff member before the anaesthetic, gladly for them as much as myself, knocked me out. On re-emerging the cyst had been lanced (oof!) and drained (grooo!) and I was home by the end of the day, sitting gingerly on the couch atop a fake fur cushion.

In 1999, off my rocker on the world's worst drug (for me, that day, at least), ecstasy, I fell off a kerb walking away from the Reading festival and broke my arm clean in two. Once more ambulanced off to A&E, I was told the injury, including extensive nerve damage, was so bad that 'you might lose your arm altogether'. Months ensued of both an orthopaedic arm brace and a flesh-coloured wrist and hand splint. It took seven months to heal, seven months of living as if underwater on super-strength painkillers, seven months of one-finger typing in a job overwhelmingly reliant on typing, of being unable to cook anything except ready meals, unable even to tie my shoelaces. Seven months of life as a helpless toddler once more, until I was eventually fixed. Again.

All of us should rejoice, every day, that this is not only the society we live in, in this country, but that we're living in it now. It wasn't so very long ago there was no NHS, and before that, no antibiotics, and before that no anaesthetic, the public enduring the kind of Victorian-era horrors my own grandparents lived through: surgeons with blood-encrusted aprons wielding rusty saws and knives at human beings so terrorised some would die from the shock alone, never mind the infection or the oceanic blood loss. It wasn't so very long ago, even in this country, we lost multiple children through not only infant mortality but the spectrum of childhood diseases, the average life expectancy in the west right up to 1850 a mere forty for men, forty-two for women. And if you were a Stone Age person, before agriculture, civilisation and any technology more advanced than a club, you'd be fortunate to make it past your teens. Which makes it all the more miraculous that any of us are here today in the first place.

Including all your friends.

11

PEDIGREE CHUMS

Friends. No one can face the tough times without their friends. Thankfully, your friends just turn up anyway because they always just turn up anyway. Your real friends, I've discovered time and time again, when you're really in trouble, just *step up*. Like a reflex, they don't think twice, they're just *there*. And in a crisis they somehow say, do, send and give you things which bind together like criss-crossed slats underneath your imperilled being until you're floating on a life raft of *them*. My pal Gavin, during his chemotherapy, had a word for this: chum-o-therapy.

We love our friends so much, in part, because they tolerate everything about us. Not always (definitely not always), but most of the time. Forgiveness, perhaps, is the key. If you're fortunate enough to have the same close friends for decades, they have seen it all, which means not only you at possibly your best – the times you're laughing together like horses – but, even more crucially, you at your very worst. The chaotically drunk you, the stressed-out you, the depressed you, the maniacal you, the furious you, the flaky you, the embarrassing you, the absent you – if work/babies/romance/stress/some existential crisis has consumed the majority of your life. But if your original bonds are strong enough, and deep enough, bonds which can bend out of shape over the years, even yield sometimes to splintering point, they will never break.

When big trouble turned up for me, my closest friends let me know, instantly and consistently: I didn't have to deal with this on my own. In fact, they wouldn't let me. Even if we didn't live in the same country. The Four of Us have lived in different cities for decades: Ev is a thirty-minute drive away in St Albans, where she's raised a family since the millennium and worked as a banking executive, already retired once and returned to freelance opportunities. Ali is five hundred miles away in Stonehaven, Scotland, also retired once already and called back to the NHS in 2021 as a much-needed Covid vaccinator. Jill has spent over thirty years three thousand miles away, in Abu Dhabi, United Arab Emirates, where she was a high-ranked midwife and raised a family, now fully retired to Ireland. As four friends go, I doubt it's possible to have four more differing characters, lifestyles, careers and domestic circumstances, but the foundations remain unshakeable.

Ev texts, when she hears I'll officially be having chemo, with a plan.

I am here with a car to drive you to any appointments 'cause you can't go to chemo on the bus!

I'm walking towards Sainsbury's and the words 'go to chemo on the bus' make me burst out blubbing. The day I text Jill with the official diagnosis, she sends several consecutive texts.

I'm not going to phone you cos I'll be blubbing and that's the last fucking thing you need. I suppose statistically one of us had to bloody fall foul of the dreaded C – shit. Anyway, I'm feeling only positivity and shall be zooming positive hugs vibes and everything else your direction.

You sound strong even though I'm sure you're bloody terrified. Treatment of breast cancer is amazing though and I know everything's going to be all right. Love you more than I could ever love a sister – you need to be okay cos I would just never get over not having P around xxx

More bawling in the street ensues.

A gift arrives from Leesa, my old *Smash Hits* pal, now five years a widow since Gavin's death. Tearing open the Amazon box, I'm peering down at a black, circular speaker. It's an Echo Dot Alexa, which I'd never thought about having before. 'Music,' reads her card, 'will see you through.'

Another day she sends a text.

Can I do anything to help? Please ask. Makes me feel useful (selfish cow that I am!) Of course you feel scared. You'd be a sociopath if you weren't. It's, quite frankly, fucking terrifying. I cannot begin to imagine the thoughts that must be racing through your head. And then trying to be positive – a lot! It's bloody tiring. Handle this how YOU want to and not how you think you should, or how others might want. If you want to retreat into a cave for a while, do it. If you want to get mad drunk and dance in the gutters like a disco goddess, then do it. Life has changed. It's OK to change with it. Xxx

She visits with her seven-year-old son for a Pizza Express soirée and presents us with another gift: a ringbinder folder full of plastic A4 sheets and post-it notes, knowing first-hand the organisation and countless hospital dates we'll have to negotiate in the coming months.

Ali sends Christmas presents. We never send each other Christmas presents. A good laugh ensues over her gifts of clothes which are exactly the sort she would wear: a floral, hippie-ish blouse, purple cosy socks and a pair of pink, heeled fluffy slippers, which say 'Audrey Hepburn' to us but definitely not to Simon. 'What's the opposite of aphrodisiac?' he scoffs. 'Naffrodisiac!?' I wear them anyway.

We spend New Year's Eve with Ev and her family and friends in St Albans, her Hogmanay a traditionally Scottish-themed affair featuring 'haggis, tatties 'n' neeps', and the 'Auld Lang

Syne' cross-body handshake hokey-cokey which always ends in disarray. New Year's Day morning traditionally brings her annual Hogmanay gift, an old-school calendar featuring landscapes of bonnie Scotland and this year is no different. Except this year everything is different.

As we're about to leave, Ev quietly slips me a large, beautifully ribboned gift bag, filled with an expensive fleecy blanket, orange-and-grey Pippi Longstocking comfy socks and a pebble inscribed with the words 'Guardian Angel'. It's to help me tolerate the cold cap: it can be so unbearable, she's researched, it helps to have something to grip onto through the lengthy, white-knuckle ride. 'I can't not have you in my life,' she says, with a rare chin wobble. Waving goodbye, I'm mascara-blind with tears as we head back to London and whatever 2020 brings. More, it will turn out, than we citizens of Earth could ever have expected.

Texts, WhatsApps, calls and gifts come in from everywhere, many with bolstering anecdotal support. Two of my oldest London pals, Gill and Trish, cheer me up like they always do. Escapees from Belfast in the still-Troubled eighties, they became my housemates in '88 and have remained forever-friends. Trish tells me a close family relative, 'had hers off [bosom] when she was about forty and is still swigging the wine at eighty-four!' Gill, known as Gilly B, a naturally non-druggy person who looked out for me during the reveller years of the early nineties, pings a text. I've just ruefully informed her of my chemo first night Cardiac Event, and she's aghast: 'Crikey! [two horror-face emojis] Just remember the doctors have given you these drugs ... not Mental Mickey!!! So you are in a safe space. Deep breaths!' The memory of Mental Mickey makes me laugh out loud, a legendary caner we knew in those reckless olden days who I used to snog, who once took so much ecstasy he had a shower in all his clothes without realising it. The nineties, eh?

Our other housemate from those olden days, Siân, another fellow *Smash Hits* musketeer, sends a Fortnum & Mason's teatime hamper – featuring a tin of shortbread with Harry and Meghan on the front, for a laugh, plus leaf tea, sweets and chocolate. She sends a text: 'God, we're all so mortal!'

Rimmy, the oldest male pal of The Four of Us since we were aged fifteen, sends a series of texts even if he is, as he says, 'speechless for once', peppering the messages with his favourite emoji, which never fails to make me laugh: the parrot. Craig, another old pal and journalist colleague (also a fellow Scot) sends a text on hearing I'm in hospital with sepsis. We'd recently worked together on an interview feature with actor Jason Watkins, a sepsis awareness-raising story highlighting the loss of Jason's two-year-old daughter Maude to the infection in 2011. No wonder, then, Craig's opening words are the highly alarmed, *'JEEEZUS FCKN MARILYN MANSON ANTICHRIST!'* Soon, I'm telling him all about the book making me laugh in hospital, the complete, five-volume *Unreliable Memoirs* of my teenage writing hero Clive James, despite listening to *'the hacking and grochels of some severely sick auld folk in the nearby Respiratory Ward'.*

'Grochels,' he texts back, of the Scottish word for clearing a phlegmy throat. *'NEVER SEEN THAT WRITTEN DOON EITHER!!! Classic. "Grochels: A Hospital Memoir", by S. Patterson.'*

We then start bantering about Paul Heaton, ex-Housemartin and Beautiful South songsmith/vocalist, who I love. *'Wibble!,'* I text, to which he replies, *'Pew Pew Barley McGrew Cuthbert WIBBLE ... PUB!'*

Who would think that one of us, at that moment, was in a hospital bed on a drip on castors with not one, but two life-threatening conditions? Which is exactly how effortless it is with your proper pals.

My family are stunned but also resolute, holding onto the word 'treatable'. Sister Jackie reassures with a Magna Carta-length list of friends, colleagues and acquaintances who've been through similar and survived. 'You know my friends, Sylv, some of them have come through it twice!' My biggest sister Liz tells me she, too, has several breast cancer-surviving friends, one of whom she plays with in a ukulele group. Even *other* people's families send support, like Ev's two sisters-in-law, who send a heart-shaped rose quartz stone, which apparently has healing vibes. It finds its home in the centre of this year's Christmas tree, alongside a strawberry, heart-shaped bauble Leesa gave us years ago in commemoration of Gavin.

I send an email to a music PR pal I've known for decades, Andy, who's not long through successful cancer treatment himself, wondering if he's any chemo tips.

'Just stay positive and get through the treatment, that was the part that kind of did it for me,' he advises. *'I just kept my head down, did everything that they required, kept exercising and trying to do all the normal shit I'd done before (within reason) ... and when you do come out the other side, as you surely will, you'll weirdly feel 'bigger' (with a different perspective on EVERYTHING) for the whole experience. I am hearing so many stories now of people's treatment changing/being modified as they progress with it, it's all getting so advanced, so am sure they'll work out what's best for you as it goes on.*

'I know the whole mention of cancer is a head-fuck beyond all things – as it must be for Simon too – but it's actually such a treatable thing now, and you will be back in the swing in no time at all, I'm sure of that. It's just gonna be an episode in your life that you'll move on from soon enough. I know it's a fucking utter cliche but my guy at the Marsden told me that staying upbeat and "forward-facing" is nearly as important in this as the very treatment itself ... you will be fine.'

Simon, too, has been sent invaluable messages from friends these last few weeks, including one of his best friends, Tom, whose wife Jamie has just been through treatment for one of the most aggressive breast cancers of them all. One partner of the sick to the other, one buddy to another, one man to another.

'It's a shocking thing but supporting each other you'll get to the end of the long road ahead,' he tells him. *'You will be in limbo and have*

a wall around you that you fear you'll never see over the top, but you will. Be positive as Sylv will need you more than ever and in turn she will support you, a team effort, and don't feel ashamed/upset to cry if that's what gets you through. It's a frustration that you can't solve "for a while" but you will both get through it. Allow yourselves to get upset and all that comes with emotions you can't control or want, face it head-on, it isn't always as bleak as it seems. After further tests you'll have a plan with the treatment, as bad as it might be, it's good, it's getting you both over the line to the next part of your life together.

'Jamie came through it with such strength and belief it was hard to think she/we went through it at all. We always treated it with contempt and laughed at it and all that goes with it. The road will seem far longer than it actually is, but be ready for some "interesting" times. Sometimes you'll want to batten down the hatches which is fine, let your chums in "as you need them", all your chums will be honoured (wrong word) to hold your hand or whatever it takes to get you two through it. You're not alone. Strength comes in several forms as you'll discover. Stay positive and allow yourselves a stumble once in a while.

'Just do what they say at the hospital and stay in love.'

I think a lot about friends right now. How lucky I am to have them. How some people have none, for a spectrum of reasons, and how pointless I would find life, if that was me. A vision appears in my mind of the last scene of *It's A Wonderful Life*, the message written in the book *Tom Sawyer*, from Clarence the angel to George Bailey, who didn't know his life was wonderful until it was taken away.

'Remember, George: no man is a failure who has friends.'

12

TEENAGE KICKS

Tuesday 17 April 1979. *Went back to school. Boring! At night went to Bell's with Sylvia to ogle at Fruity and Andy.*

Wednesday 18 April 1979. *Ian chucked Sylvia. She was seek. Did nothing at Bell's. Then went to Perthshire Club. It was crap.*

Friday 20 April 1979. *Police Disco with Sylv. Fantastic! I did a lot of grooving and freaking out. Got lots of dances. Got a moonie from* [idiotic nickname] *Plan 80!*

We've newly turned fourteen years of age and we're still never in, the evidence of our whereabouts, and with-whom-abouts, conscientiously collated in Ali's teenage diaries from 1979 to 1983. What strikes me most, as I read them today, is the innocence, energy and romantic belief in the face of endless rebuffal; and how much music and dancing mattered; and the constant evidence of the scattergun intensity we all endure through the bedlam of adolescence. I was always 'seek' (Scottish for 'sick') when some random boy wasn't interested, but I cast my net, as her diaries continuously assure me, as wide as the North Sea.

By early 1980, we weren't just 'out' in the open, we were forever out in the pubs, playing darts and pool with nineteen-year-old boys (some actually men in their early twenties), who assumed we were, somehow, twenty-year-old women. When 'our' lads were getting off with other girls, a vigilant Ali would document the supposed betrayal and our indignant dual reaction: *'Went to Sylv's and had fags because we were absolutely pissed off.'* Mostly, though, they protected us, a comedy collective we'd call The Troops, their central character, Rimmy, keeping vigilant eyes around the kids they called 'the schoolies'.

Our favourite pub was The Grill, tucked away down a narrow alleyway in central Perth (the terrifyingly titled Fleshers Vennel), a windowless, ground-floor dungeon with minimal lighting where the bar staff, perhaps, couldn't see how young we were (more likely didn't care). Here, the post-punk insurgence thundered from the wall-mounted jukebox (The Jam, PiL, Specials, Bauhaus, Magazine, Gang of Four), nights funded by saved-up school dinner money and our jobs in Bell's Sports Centre. We'd make a half-cider last an hour and buy ten More cigarettes between us, the thin brown cigarillos which made us feel *terribly* sophisticated. Our favourite club was St Albans on a Friday night, established in '79 in the mod revival uprising throughout Britain's provinces, where I took to wearing four-inch-long miniskirts and six-inch stilettos I could not walk one yard in today. With free entry before 9 p.m., we'd sidle in at 8.45, have another half-cider and dance all night pretending we were the cast of *Quadrophenia*, all sixties' moves and handmade clothes, often from gaudy old curtains – a dancefloor of teenagers losing their minds to The Beat, The Selecter, Madness and especially The Who, guffaws exchanged over the lyrics in '5.15', 'Girls of fifteen, sexually knowing!' Skinny-tied, mod-u-like mannequins Secret Affair's immortal one-hit-wonder 'Time For Action' saw arms in the air like wind-blown triffids – 'Oi! Oi! Oi!' – which always erupted into the communal chant, 'We are the mods! We are the mods! We are, we are, we are the mods!' We were the mods, then.

In March 1980 we both turned fifteen.

*

Friday 7 March 1980. *Went down town after school for Sylv's birthday present. I got her £4.25 Cavale Rust Eyeshadow* and 20 More, 77p. At night altered dress for tomorrow night. Went out at 9.30 to the Rugby Club Disco. It was quite good.*

In summer 1980 I temporarily ruined *everything* by winning a local secondary schools essay competition run by the 1917-established Perth Rotary Club (subject: My Chosen Career), writing fantasy capers about the life of a sports journalist, despite knowing nothing about any form of journalism. Disastrously for me, though, the four winners across four schools were assembled and photographed for the local newspapers, my newly peroxide blonde, elfin-cropped hair beaming out from the group photo like a keyboard player in a synth-pop band amusingly dressed up as a schoolgirl. The message was clear: 'HELLO PUBS AND CLUBS OF PERTH I AM FIFTEEN YEARS OF AGE AND DRINKING IN YOUR ESTABLISHMENT ILLEGALLY.' Duly rumbled, myself and Ali blithely turned up to our usual saloons – The Grill, St Albans, The Cavern, the Sally (Salutation Hotel, which held a club night known as Scandals) – to be met with either requests for proof of age we did not possess, or the raising of a doorman/publican's arm and the unambiguous instruction, 'OUT.'

Saturday 12 July 1980. *Went to Grill then Scandals. Sylv got in but after one hr ten mins she was asked for proof of age and kicked out*

---

*When I read this diary entry, I felt certain I still had this eyeshadow. I knew it was antique, that it came from the eighties and I always thought it was my sister Jackie's. In 1980, £4.25 was a lot of money (worth £19.42 today, inflation fans). If I still wore eyeshadow, which I don't, I don't think I'd pay £4.25 for one *now*. Yes: rummaging around in my circular tin of old and emergency make-up, it's there: a stylish, stand-up glass bottle, the colour of rust, the words 'Faberge', 'Cavale' and 'Shimmer Shadow' etched on the front in thin, white lettering. Opening the white, square lid I peer inside and there's still a centimetre of rust eyeshadow nestled at the bottom, forty-two years later. Cherish something enough, it seems, and you'll keep it for ever.

and banned for life. We went to the Shanghai afterwards [frequently visited, post-club chip shop] *and walked up the road with Alan Morrison. Totally pissed off.*

Undaunted, the very next day we found a new disco which *would* let us in, The Wheel Inn, a nightclub in a hotel on the road to nearby Scone.

Sunday 13 July 1980. *Went to the Wheel Inn at night. It was magic. FANTASTIC.*

Within just five months, in time for Hogmanay, we were back in even more pubs than ever, staying out 'til six in the morning.

By now, we'd both gravitated to better-paid jobs than the café counter in Bell's; Ali in a bakery, me the chief dish-washer in Perth police station. I'd done many illegal things by then (booze, fags, occasional puffs on a spliff), so this appointment made me chuckle, the job made bearable by a small radio/cassette player nestled inside the police station kitchen. Singing amongst the steamy machines, I'd blare the albums of Killing Joke, The Psychedelic Furs and Iggy Pop, albums taped from the vinyl collections of our older boy buddies, keenly contributing to the 'home taping is killing music' era, just as the Sony Walkman swung into technological view.

At sixteen I was, in my head, some kind of revolutionary, as befitted those revolutionary times; the late seventies/early eighties era was one of culture's most enduringly vibrant – sonically, visually, politically – from post-punk's esoteric clanging to the party-hard two-tone titans to the ghoulish goths to the posturing new romantics to the art school dreamers and foppish indie schemers. The culture was dynamic on all levels, defined by diverse musical dynamism, alternative comedy, feminism, gay liberation, CND marches and The Young People Versus Margaret Thatcher. Night-time Radio 1 soundtracked The Revolution via three pivotal spirits: John Peel, Janice Long and Annie Nightingale. This trio would be more responsible for creating the lifelong values of Britain's

Generation X than any government or institution could ever hope to be. We were ideologically pure, our principles black-and-white, with a dominant music press which consolidated everything. I was a music magazine obsessive, a devoted apostle of *Sounds*, *NME*, *Record Mirror* and *Smash Hits*, with sprout-fringed 1981 hair, a politically indignant, republican renegade who, on 29 July 1981 – the day of Prince Charles and Lady Di's wedding – hatched a plot with Rimmy and various Troops to stage a monarchy-toppling protest. In a righteous huff at the Union Jack bunting festooned around the pubs of Perth, we strode up to Kinnoull Hill (a cliffside walk overlooking the Dundee Road and infamous suicide spot), smoked dope and giggled our heads off. The following day, somehow, the monarchy had failed to fall.

This was the year I lost my virginity, on a school skiing holiday featuring The Four of Us, to Monte Bondone, Italy.

Saturday 4 April 1981. *Skiing was brill. Got suntan on face. At night went to disco. Sylv got off with an Iti* [pronounced 'aye-tie', as Italians were routinely known, a now derogatory term which would doubtless see Ali's diaries cancelled in every university curriculum in the land].

His name was Walter, and he was *gorgeous*, liquid-brown eyes and tantalising lips, a cartoon pretty face encircled in a mane of tumbling dark brown curls. We were in his car, halfway up a mountain, having drunk a bottle of Pernod between us, when the snogging turned the windows, and our heads, irretrievably steamy. This was *it*, I knew. I was willing. From somewhere amid the steam he produced a condom. 'It is all right?' he beseeched, all blinkless Bambi eyes, possibly the only words of English he knew (and, evidently, needed to know). I nodded. I'd been sixteen for a whole month and he really *was* so irresistibly attractive. It was all over in two minutes. He drove me a few hundred yards back down the mountain, stopped at a crossroads and indicated this was where I got out, without so much as a suggestion of a sheepish look on his smouldering Italian face. On I trudged back to the chalet, alone, deflowered, bewildered, on the Pernod, halfway up a snowy Italian mountainside, vaguely wandering towards a village I could not remember the name of. (And we worry about 'ver kids' of today.)

On we caroused, never in, the nights we weren't out dancing – say, a Wednesday – spent in a pub called Ramekins which projector-screened the latest films (*Raging Bull, The Jazz Singer, Gregory's Girl, Herbie Goes Bananas*).

I made my first and final attempt to be the singer of a band, 'auditioning' as frontwoman of a group I knew nothing about. The audition was held in one of Perth's grandly stern old churches. Vibrating with nerves, I drank three pints of Carlsberg Special, with lime, wobbled into the church, clattered onto the stage, approached the microphone and bawled, in political indignation, 'Maggie! Maggiieeeeee! Nooooooo!' before running back out the door. The reign of The Clash continued, uncontested by the likes of me.

Soon, a new club had replaced St Albans – the Banana Club: Perth's post-punk/indie mecca, DJ'd by a friend of Rimmy's, John McKeand. Briefly, John became my boyfriend, soon travelling four hundred miles with me to see Echo And The Bunnymen at the Hammersmith Palais, London, the same year I began wearing a gentleman's overcoat to school exactly like Bunnymen frontman Ian McCulloch's, with a noble belief in the look and mindset of the singular 'individual'.

At seventeen I temporarily lost Ali to her first proper boyfriend, a madman whose name she can barely say to this day. He'd meet her every day after school, sometimes at lunchtime too, constantly phone her at home in the evening (making sure she was in). She loved him though, and learned, ultimately, how to spot the kind of wrong 'un who (as Kylie once so memorably put it), 'is attracted to the birds of paradise and then they put you in a box and your colours fade'. Nonetheless, we'd still always watch *Top of the Pops* together, followed by the *Kenny Everett Television Show* and afterwards she'd write in her diary, '*had a good laugh with Sylv*'. Very occasionally, we'd sneak a night out.

Friday 19 February 1982. *Went to school. At night went out with Sylv. Went to Jim's. Had four joints. Totally wrecked. Then went to Cave and Grill. Totally pissed. Went home at 12.30. Had brilliant night.*

Otherwise, the diary entry for my seventeenth birthday says it all:

Monday 8 March 1982. *Sylv's birthday. School. At night went to Sylv's for a wee while.* [Madman] *phoned. Got Meatloaf record. Washed hair and had a bath. Went to bed early.*

We turned eighteen and everything changed as jobs turned up and locations began to shift, as life's tectonic plates always will.

Tuesday 8 March 1983. *Sylv's birthday. Have been accepted for nursing. I start August this year. Yippee!*

Tuesday 24 May 1983. *Sylv came round to tell me about her job.* Watched the film Some Like It Hot. *Really funny.*

Wednesday 25 May 1983. *LEAVE SCHOOL!!*

The next big adventure, of adulthood, had begun.

13

MY FUNNY VALENTINE

I've become the most boring bastard on Earth. Light years away from the cavorting teenager with the vertical hair, bouncing off the walls in The Grill. I'm so bored *with myself.* At home, after the sepsis incarceration, all life consists of is waiting for the next poisoning, enduring the greatest level of extreme boredom I have ever known.

Serious illness does this to you, as you steadily morph into a one-note, human monotone of insularity and self-absorption, which you would loathe in anyone else. Already this illness and the treatment of it is all I talk about, think about, am asked about and know about. Everything else has disappeared, every other aspect of life before, or in the future, *all gone*, or at least suspended, perhaps in formaldehyde, like Damien Hirst's shark, the one he called *The Physical Impossibility of Death in the Mind of Someone Living*, a title which suddenly makes no sense to me whatsoever.

After a week's postponement, Chemo 2 happens, and back home things deteriorate. I'm bone-chilled again, even with three layers on, including my biggest, woolliest jumper, with the heating on full blast. Schlepping round the flat I see a vision in the full-length living-room mirror, of a wounded yeti, shoulders slumped, zero makeup, the worst of clothes, bedraggled hair (weakened follicles mean you're advised to wash it sparingly, every four days at most), appearing ten years older than I was one month ago. Sleepless nights include a racing heartbeat, the day brings much Bathroom Activity and I've yet to start work on the Amy book: Tyler has also been waylaid, thwarted by his own personal dramas.

The days are spent aimlessly, attempting to gee myself up with the jokes of Clive James, but there's nothing to look forward to, no chance of respite, fed up, without purpose. I've been sick or weird or cold or sore or hospitalised for the last five weeks. Five weeks ... *is that all?!*

The mouth ulcers return, some erupting on the tongue, some along the gums, a large patch on my inside right cheek resembling a soft-centred Danish pastry. It sounds so namby-pamby – 'I've a sore mouth, boo hoo!' – but this pain is intense, deep inside the bones of the gums, like the after-effects of root canal surgery. Sometimes, it feels like the *middle* of root canal surgery ... in 1892 ... before anaesthetic was invented. Life becomes existence in a waiting room, waiting-waiting-waiting for all this to go away. My temperature is climbing, a call to the chemo ward instructing I must now come in for a blood test. *Oh puh-lease, no.*

Nadia greets me with gentle concern. Extracting blood is a problem, as ever, but she manages the requisite half-an-armful. I feel better already, enveloped by the comforting familiarity of this no longer alien environment, knowing the staff in here are the only ones who can fix me, who can make this madness, even temporarily, go away. No harm, I'm certain, can befall me in here, I don't have to make decisions about how ill I am, about how many times I should take my temperature, or have any opinions at all. Nadia tells me it's normal to feel this cold, a side effect of the E half of the EC chemo (the lengthily titled epirubicin cyclophosphaminde). Smiling rumly on the inside, this conjures thoughts of the 1990s, the most culturally carefree decade I've yet lived through; the raves and the dancing and the smiley faces, when the only E poisoning my body was half a tab of ecstasy in the 'healing' fields of Glastonbury.

Today is 14 February, Valentine's Day. It happens to be the day Simon is also called to a clinic, a bothersome groin taking him to a specialist outpatients' in east London where he's being felt up, as we speak, for testicular cancer. Rarely a sick man, and 'inspired' by my early diagnosis, it's the first time he's ever presented himself to medics for anything this potentially serious. For weeks I've been beseeching the universe: spare him, spare him, spare him ... not both of us crocked by chemo, surely, at exactly the same time.

The blood results are in: I'm diagnosed with neutropenic sepsis once again and burst into shocked, hot-faced tears. The self-administered white-blood-cell stimulus injections haven't worked and the chemo is working too well: it's wiping out all the cells it should be wiping out, but it's also wiping me out, the classic baby-out-with-the-bath-water scenario. It's now 1.45 p.m. and all there is left on the lunch trolley is a rejected falafel wrap. So, when Simon turns up to see me, having had his scrotum gelled and fondled by a female stranger with an ultrasound wand, we share the falafel wrap, our meal together on this special day in 2020. Happy Valentine's Day, my love.

I'm imprisoned once again, in a quarantined side room, this time affiliated to the cardiac ward. The room has no loo, so I'm given a personal commode, the first time in my life I've ever used one, for which I am grateful. Otherwise, I'd have to use the loo round the corner, in a ward which is populated by rows of pale, sunken-cheeked souls who appear to be dead already. The light is even bleaker than in the last room, the windows frosted, blocking out even the faintest daylight, the squares overhead emanating a gloomy grey, as if my life is now lived in permanent, Dickensian fog.

The following day Simon brings a new lamp, seven pounds

from Argos. I've been fitted with a heart monitor for forty-eight hours, a constellation of pads, wires and a digital box now stuck to my body, making sleep even less likely than it was already. That evening, watching BBC News 24 on my phone, shocking news arrives of the suicide of *Love Island* presenter Caroline Flack. If sleep was problematic before, now it becomes impossible, I'm tormented, can't stop thinking about how Fame, these days, Is Hell.

Since the mid-eighties I've seen fame up close, in all its warped, devious, delusional forms, though it's often simultaneously funny, a ludicrously privileged non-reality which has been skewing lives since the dawn of the public figure. While scandal, rumour, gossip and bitching have existed for ever, ruthless tabloid tyranny and social media have not, and that fittingly blood-red, A-list carpet is piled ever higher with the bodies of the broken, drunk, drugged, bankrupt, scandalised and suicidal famous.

Sitting in my hospital bed, a parade of past magazine interviews flash by and I count on one hand the global stars I've encountered who are not only good at fame but seemingly actively enjoy it. Bono. Noel Gallagher. Catherine Zeta Jones. George Clooney (even if he hung up on me in 2008 after a cheeky *Glamour*-magazine-shaped query as to the cohabiting status of his latest girlfriend). And Jennifer Aniston who, back in 2011, dealt with her then-permanent position on the cover of the *National Enquirer*, America's shameless megaphone of made-up blather, with impressive, good-natured grace. I talked to her on the phone and also wrote around a buy-in interview, where she mused on her feelings about fame.

'Fame is an odd beast,' she confirmed. 'Because there's nothing real about it. You're only one person like everybody else and yet you're projected as almost superhuman. Cameras in your face, lies, rumours, there's so much that's taken or wanted.' Sometimes, she added, even *she* woke up and thought, 'I don't know if I'm as big as this beast.'

But the majority of the super-famous seem to merely tolerate fame as an unfortunate occupational side effect. I remember Zac Efron, the sometime most famous young man on Earth through the *High School Musical* era of the noughties who, while filming in Canada aged twenty-two, found the sight of empty sidewalks not thronging with paparazzi the most 'beautiful!' sight he'd ever seen. 'I cherish all the ordinary things in my life,' he stressed and called the celebrity that surrounded him 'The Madness'.

Back in 1998, then thirty-nine-year-old Madonna also pondered the illusory nature of fame. 'Fame,' she decided, 'is what everybody else puts on you, it's their own fantasy, nothing to do with me at all. Fascinating, really.'

This stirred another memory, of being in a countryside studio barn in 2018 interviewing Matty Healy, frontman with UK electro-indie pop scamps The 1975. He was talking about their 'hardcore, crazy fans' – millions of them – in his personal world of extreme fame. Two weeks beforehand, when I took the assignment, happy to be delving into a contemporary pop phenomenon, I wouldn't have known Matty Healy if he'd turned up on my doorstep offering a free busk of his previous No. 1 album, which I also did not know. So, to me, he wasn't famous at all. After all these years sharing space with the exceptionally famous, it felt like a revelation: people really *are* only famous if you, personally, think they are; their fame really *does* exist only in your own head. Exactly as Madonna said.

Fame, though, for years, hasn't looked like much fun for anyone. Where a star's fame, at least initially, was once predominantly celebrated, today it's more readily mercilessly scorned, since the rise of all-pervasive, twenty-first-century Celebrity Culture and its two distinct offshoots: being-famous-for-being-famous and reality TV, bringing their own specific by-product, the devaluing of fame. The 2000s gave us a gleefully cut-throat tabloid culture, the one which conspired to break the spirit of Amy Winehouse in the UK and Britney Spears in the US. The fate of those two young women perhaps illustrates best why our pop stars, today, are the least chaotic in history, ever mindful of their mental health. The tabloids, meanwhile, are marginally less toxic, though hardly in their coverage of Caroline Flack, possibly their most recent showbiz nadir.

Back in 2007, even the swaggering Liam Gallagher, as Oasis began to implode, spent the first of our two interviews with an overcoat zipped up to his chin and a manbag wedged to his lap, as if acting as a psychic shield. I wondered that year if he, as a person, ever felt vulnerable in any way? 'You're vulnerable,' he coolly told me, his unblinking blue eyes fixed straight ahead, 'every time you open your fookin' mouth.' And this was before the rise of social media, the dominance of which, alongside 'clickbait', has ignited permanent paranoia, stars tolerating interviews today (if they grant them at all) through a filter of suspicion and vigilant self-censorship. No wonder.

Caroline Flack was a professional TV presenter, shepherding the ordinary beautiful young people through the *Love Island* experience. She'd known depression throughout her life, her arrest and accusation of assaulting her boyfriend trumpeted across the triumphant UK tabloids for weeks, wilfully feeding vicious online abuse. 'To the press, the newspapers, who create clickbait, who demonise and tear down success, we've had enough,' announced Caroline's buddy Laura Whitmore on her BBC Radio 5 Live show within hours of the dreadful news of her death. 'I've seen journalists and Twitter warriors talk of this tragedy and they themselves twisted what the truth is,' she carried on. 'Your words affect people. To paparazzi and tabloids looking for a cheap sell, to trolls hiding behind a keyboard, enough.'

For Caroline Flack and so many more, fame and fragile mental health is a deadly combination. Caroline surely partly died of shame. Of embarrassment. Of being judged. Or how she perceived she was being judged, by the same brutalising media forces we've been saying 'enough' to, now, for years. Shame on them. Shame on a society which encourages them. *Shame on us.*

Sleepless nights continue: lights unapologetically click on at 2 a.m. for blood pressure, then 4 a.m. for antibiotic drip-bag change, then 5 a.m. for a blood test. Since 4 a.m. someone has been in deep distress, shouting, 'Nurse!' and 'Help!' It's hugely upsetting and hugely annoying, and I can't believe I feel annoyed: this is surely someone's parent, or grandparent, or someone years younger than I am, very likely on their deathbed.

At 6 a.m., even before the morning porridge arrives (from the 1970s), a bowel twitch occurs, the first 'movement' in forty-eight hours. You can't not see the result, squatting inside the commode pan, an *enormous*, solid circular mound, with a perfectly tapering tail. It will have to sit there, under the pan lid, under copious, concealing toilet paper, until professionally removed. A nurse arrives, removes the brim-full pan and I'm humiliated once again, like living through The Worst Glastonbury Ever. I apologise, mortified.

'It is fine!' she breezes. 'There are no complaints.'

The inside of my right cheek is now so ravaged with ulcerated sores it looks like the health warning on a packet of cigarettes. Worse, I'm running out of Difflam mouthwash, distracting myself by watching snooker highlights and reading more tormenting headlines about Caroline Flack. It's just before dawn and I'm crushed with exhaustion, mulling this new reality: how can it be that this, now, is my life? There's nothing in it but hospital, medication, soreness and misery. As grateful as I am to be here. All I have is time, but it's time warped by pain, fatigue and worry. I'd thought having all this time would be a luxury, you'd just read amazing books all day but it's not possible, reading takes full engagement, effort, and I don't have the energy or the focus. I need something beamed towards me, a blanket of distraction, like sport. I'm too tired to even write a text properly.

I've been in bed so long my backside is developing the sores of a bedbound ninety-five-year-old. I can still hear the shouter next door, yelling, 'Oh god!', hacking and convulsing in fear and agony. It's been going on for the last three hours, like being in a prison where the next door inmate has gone clinically insane. Maybe this, I'm now thinking, is what The End will be like for all of us, if we're lucky enough to even have a deathbed. I stare at the commode in the corner of my room, which has had no pan in it for over half an hour. Danger! Danger!

Fifteen minutes later, the nurse returns with the emptied pan, in silence, and leaves again in silence. She's exhausted: all the nurses have listened to the shouting all night, too.

My veins are still on strike. I was to have a 'port' fitted, a state-of-the-art circular gizmo surgically positioned under the skin near the collar bone where all treatments can flow, meaning no more cannula calamities. And now, because of sepsis, it must be postponed. The head chemo nurse Renée comes to visit. She's so kind I crumble, openly crying, and she gives me a rib-crusher hug, as she reassures me over and over: 'You will get better! And this treatment will work! And you will recover!'

I remind myself, forcefully, this is not a terminal diagnosis. You will get back to life, eventually.

A nurse arrives to takes notes on bathroom activities. Urine. *Tick.* Bowel movement. *Tick.* Because I've had a movement she whips her phone out and scrolls to a page where I'm to choose the closest version from a chart of the spectrum of human faeces. There's nothing on that chart resembling the whopper which arrived this morning.

On another morning a nurse arrives with an antibiotic, the one known as 'the stingy one' and administers, through the cannula jabbed in the crook of my arm, the 'flush' of tube-clearing saline.

Aiiieeeee! It's like an injection of molten lava. She tries again, several times – lava! lava! – before declaring the cannula line bust. It was feeding into tissue, not vein. I need a new one. Again.

A full hour later another nurse arrives, jabs a new line, shouts, 'I forgot the gauze!', bolts out of the room and leaves me with a huge needle and container full of blood dangling out of a vein. Ali rings and I'm boo-hoo-hooing all over again.

I'm there for four more nights. The sleep deprivation intensifies, not only because of the guttural howls of the traumatised or the two-hourly visits for obs, but the sound of the treatment saving my life. The digital feeder pump is louder than ever, a monotonous metronome – pssssst ... psssst ... psssst ... – rhythmic, mechanical, relentless. It also sounds archaic, like a throwback from the industrial age and, not for the first time, I think: In decades to come, all this will seem (sort of) laughable, early twenty-first-century cancer treatment the equivalent of the SMASH adverts from the 1970s, where the robots on the spaceship cackle over the folly of the olden human ways: 'They peeled it with their metal knives!'

This time, I'm given no injections to speed the production of white blood cells. Renée has explained: Dr Bridger needs to know if my body can produce them itself. Right now, it can't or only very slowly. So I'm staying at least another day. Possibly, at this rate, till Easter.

One day a nurse wheels in with the obs machine, sees my Argos lamp blazing on the bedside table and announces, 'You are living like a princess! In here, with your lamp, all to yourself ...'

'I'd rather be living under a bridge and be free!'

She doesn't reply, her eyes wide over her mask. I hope she's smiling too.

I think about my dad on his deathbed in 1989, chained up to a drip much like I am today, his final days spent succumbing to this dreadful disease I'm now experiencing myself. It was a bowel cancer diagnosis my family hid from me for over a year, thinking I wouldn't be able to cope; in those days cancer was the unspeakable, as if somehow a personal shame, referred to only as 'the C word'. (Mind you, that decade, they didn't even tell me the family cat had been dead for six months, until I visited, wondering out loud, 'Where's Bubbles?') I only knew something was wrong with Dad on a visit home, driving together through town, when he stopped the car abruptly and rushed into a public toilet. When he came back, I could tell he'd been humiliated. The next time I saw him he was in hospital, this gracious, capable, once Sean-Connery-sized man now a spindle-limbed skeleton, his last words to me some advice for his wayward youngest child.

'For God's sake Sylvia, look after your health, you can't beat it.'

I'd just turned twenty-four, he was sixty-nine and, of course, he was absolutely right. Two decades followed of smoking, drinking and dancing, ever reaching for Noel Gallagher's description of the purpose of Oasis, to 'celebrate the euphoria of life', as if I would, somehow, as the Oasis song promised, live forever. I didn't listen to my dad then, but I hear him loud and clear today. Wellness is paradise. Without health we have nothing. As soon as you're sick, on any level – be it a cold, a broken arm, anywhere on the spectrum of disease, both physical and mental – all you want is your old life back. The normal one, that 'boring' one, the one you didn't fully realise was everything you'll ever need, brimful of everyday banality.

News arrives of the death of maverick DJ Andy Weatherall, producer of Primal Scream's era defining *Screamadelica* in 1991. Gone at fifty-six from a blood clot, a sudden pulmonary embolism. It's a bona-fide shocker, my generation of The Greats being picked off one by one, already. I know, now, I want to live to be *properly* ancient. What would it be like, still laughing, maybe even dancing, at a hundred, with the friends you've been laughing and dancing with for, ooh, not far off the full century?

Finally, I'm discharged, suddenly packing up in a frenzy while two nurses are stripping my bed already, preparing for the next poor soul's misadventure in sleep deprivation. Back home, the TV news tells me the world has imploded: it's February 2020 and there's flooding all over the country, farmers doomed, Wales and north Yorkshire underwater, Caroline Flack still dead, nine people murdered in a shisha shop in Germany, a seventy-year-old man stabbed in the neck in a central mosque, the sentencing of the New Zealand, Tinder date-rapist killer of Grace Millane ... out here, it's a vale of tears. A consultant rings with results of Simon's ultrasound: his problem is a common benign cyst, he doesn't have testicular cancer. My personal world, at least, slots back on its axis. Temporarily.

14

BACK ON THE CHAIN GANG

Fantastically organised admin skills continue to dominate reality as I now know it. Oh, *the admin*. Which only reinforces your new status as the most boring bastard on Earth. A reality filled with appointments and phone calls and consultations and treatments and follow-up appointments which means, to keep track of where you're supposed to be and when and with whom and why, you must become your own personal illness secretary. To this end, there's now a *second* calendar on the kitchen wall, a Hospital Calendar, a free 2020 one from BBC *Springwatch* featuring stunning scenes of wildlife, where all forthcoming appointments are logged.

The kitchen table now hosts my Cancer Treatment Record Book, an admin tool from the chemo suite, with pages of side-effect notes to be registered, featuring rows of suggested ailments alongside increasingly darkening circles which you must tick, documenting your symptoms from 'mild' to 'severe': *Abnormal temperature* (note: 'freezing!'), *Bleeding and bruising* ('nosebleeds'), *Sore mouth* ('brutal, scalded throat'), *Pain* ('gums, brushing teeth brutal'), *Constipation* ('yes'), *Mood* ('very fed up at sepsis happening again').

I also have a personal diary, a pink Taylor Swift 2020 promo freebie, with a dreamy photo of the gifted pop giraffe on the cover below the word '*Lover*' (her 2019 album). So now I am the kind of person who is writing in a Taylor Swift diary such notable daily activities as: 'Bowels move!' 'All pills taken.' 'Awake 2 a.m.' 'Awake 3.15 a.m.' 'Bit spaced out. Can't take loud noises.' 'Raw gums, man!' 'Proper pain all over mouth.' 'No sleep, Smokey Robinson "Tracks Of My Tears" blaring in head all night.' 'Totally pissed off now, no respite from feeling dreadful.' 'Hospital.' 'Acute ward.' 'Hell.' Surely not what Swift would've wanted.

Suddenly, there's progress. 'Mouth: increments of improvement.' Then: 'Massive mouth improvement at last!' For ten full days I'm visited by the miracle of normality. The mouth pain is barely detectable, all foods are consumable, I'm not bone-chilled or fevered, even if sleep is still broken. I see my friends in the pub and *laugh*. Even if – with Chemo 3 given the go-ahead – I know this holiday in normality will shortly end.

Before that, I can finally be fitted with the treatment port at a different hospital in central London. The surgeon is a comedy medic who looks like toothsome Liverpool FC manager Jurgen 'Clippity' Klopp. He makes jokes about a starter shot of anaesthetic feeling like 'a lovely gin 'n' tonic!' Back home wearing a bulky, padded dressing it's impossible to sleep for a new reason: there's an alien piece of hardware wedged inside my body which includes a temporary needle. Lying on my right side, which I normally do, is agony. Instead, I must lie face up like Tutankhamun's mummy. When I'm up, I'm shambling around at forty-five degrees like the victim of an overnight stroke.

But at least I'm finally back at work.

In early March, I begin the Amy Winehouse book. My ghostwriting task takes discipline and copious time, guiding Tyler through his lifetime's friendship with the human whirlwind Winehouse, walking up and down the balcony outside our flat, phone wedged to my ear, for up to three hours at a time (it will take around sixty hours of interviews altogether). It's one hell of a story.

The relief of being physically and mentally able to work is huge.

Hearing, transcribing and editing the dam-busting torrents of emotion from Tyler proves an agreeably time-consuming and sanity-saving project, giving me a surge of energy, positivity and belief. We all need a purpose in life. Maybe even more so when we're ill. Because otherwise we're just *ill*. Work makes me feel like the person I used to be, finally thinking and talking about something other than being ill and having my life turned into an unemployed person's perpetual walk in the park.

Simultaneously, though, for the first time in my working life I'm beginning to see the appeal of stopping. Because so many friends, the ones who are financially stable, are stopping. The other three of The Four of Us are either close to full retirement or there already, as is Rimmy. I've always known I'll be the only one of my inner circle who can never retire, because I can't afford to. Simon is the same. It's the biggest price of the 'freedom' I've coveted above all else. A freedom which has meant I have no financial security and there are no sums pending in the future, either, through inheritance, or nestling pension. And now I'm watching my buddies and acquaintances, one after the other, reap the rewards of a lifetime of financial common sense and job stability in careers as alien to me as mine has been to them. Some of them have had jobs their whole lives they've loathed. I've always loved my job. And if you love your job, I've always thought, why would you stop? But music journalism isn't the job it used to be. It doesn't really *exist* any more, gone the way of town criers, whistling milkmen and bus conductors. All of us who've seen our livelihoods decimated by technology in recent years must, therefore, in the Darwinian way, adapt or die. But if I had the choice, which is the very best thing money can buy, I'm beginning to think I *would*. Just stop.

These days, I'm sure I could easily fill my time, hanging out with Simon, with friends, visiting family, days happily spent walking, reading and podcast listening and, in the ideal scenario, with travelling through the grand cities of Europe, learning, nourishing all the senses through culture, food, history, geography, architectural splendour and the intoxicating exposure to different kinds of people. But you can only do all of that when you have money.

I rerun in my mind the conversation I had back in the nineties with Shaun Ryder, seated on villa porch steps in Jamaica, where he was making a video with his post-Happy Mondays group Black Grape. I asked him a question, taken from a phrase I'd heard which intrigued me at the time: *What do you think about the phrase, 'You are free to do whatever you like, you need only face the consequences'?*

'I've never been free to do what I like,' he mused, sipping from a bottle of Guinness. 'What I wanted to do was just live and be happy and always have nice clothes and do nothing. But I can't 'cos I've got no dough. At the end of the day, if I was born into money, I wouldn't do a fookin' *stroke*. Not for commercial gain. I might scribble in a diary about me last ninety-seven years as a complete sail-in-the-seas opium-smoking arsehole. Or I might've tried to invent penicillin, that'd be cool. But I can't do nothing, 'cos I'm a pirate.'

I asked him what he thought life was for, which he responded to after several minutes' pause.

'To explore,' he concluded. 'Definitely. That's what it's all about, man, go forth and explore.'

Work, then, wasn't it. And it never is, especially the older we become. Especially when we're facing the end of our lives, as we're told over and over by those who spend their own working lives tending to the dying. Back in 2012, the Australian writer and sometime carer Bronnie Ware published the international bestseller *The Top Five Regrets of the Dying*, which cited the second-biggest regret as, 'I wish I hadn't worked so hard.' Number 1 was: 'I wish I'd had the courage to live a life true to myself, not the life others expected of me.' Which can often mean, of course, a life defined by the job you didn't want to do, but you did because it was expected of you.

Through the eighties, nineties and into the early 2000s I gave my every waking second to work, obsessively so, often working through the night, almost never going on holiday, making the two common mistakes which befall so many freelancers: never saying 'No' (because you think you might never work in this town again) and believing 'I am what I do' (the mindset of many so-called creatives). It's a perilous condition, submerging self-worth and self-esteem inside a catastrophically unstable domain, where how good you feel about yourself is contingent on someone else's opinion (which is understandable, given that, if the someone else who is employing you thinks you're hopeless, you really *will* never work in this town again).

Here in my mid-fifties, though, I realise why this is the age when many, if they can, begin eyeing up the eject button. You've only so much energy left and you'd rather spend it elsewhere. Would I really want to keep working till I drop? Dying of an actual cardiac event aged seventy-nine, mid-descriptive musing on whatever technology I don't understand this week, found slumped over the computer, an indentation in my cheek the shape of the 'cmd' button on a Mac keyboard?

But the chances are, as the still-busy Shaun Ryder knows, if you've got no dough, you've got no choice. So slumped over the computer at seventy-nine it is, then, if I even make it that far (which is doubtful). And it's all your fault, the Righteous Teenage Revolutionary.

The month I finally get back to work, however, one subject begins to dominate our twenty-four-hour rolling news, which makes me even more grateful to have work to do and work I can do at home.

'Of course,' said Dr Bridger during our last consultation, 'if this coronavirus coming in from China gets any worse, we're all in trouble ...'

15

IT'S OH SO QUIET

Chemo 3 sees the suite staff gather round to observe my port and coo as if it's a new-born child or a very expensive sports car.

'Ooh, you've got a posh one!'

They can see its contours clearly under the skin, a circular plastic pod with three protruding points, all the better to locate the middle section where an incoming needle will be lodged. In very overweight people, they can't see the port properly, it's lost under layers of fatty skin so they're aiming the needle blind, a shot in the dark. Mine is therefore 'excellent!' It works perfectly: the needle is inserted through the skin, into the port, a saline flush goes in, blood comes out, no pain whatsoever, a tube is attached, the drip bag of chemo goes up on the pole with the castors and treatment begins. This thing is a miracle. And if I was an American without robust healthcare, it would've cost $2,200 to have it fitted and the same to have it taken out again. It is the NHS, in fact, which is the miracle. And now it has to deal with a global pandemic.

Two days later on 7 March 2020, two deaths from Coronavirus are recorded in the UK and 164 positive tests. Soon, it's the only news topic on Earth. Philosophical discourse floods the rolling news, fevered talk everywhere on how this will change us, change society, change politics, change working lives and the way we all live for ever. As businesses begin to shut down and a torpedo heads for the global economy, it feels like the planet has stopped *itself* turning. As if the world knew it was spinning too fast and shut itself down, to save itself from *us*. Look at yourselves, it seems to be saying: *look* at what you've become.

Piers Morgan on *Good Morning Britain* is having the time of his life, shouting at politicians and frothing over rich people supposedly buying their own ventilators. A talking head pipes in with The Big Picture: 'I think there's now a realisation that we all want the same things, to protect each other, solidarity, have enough to survive. We need measures in place to make sure we can achieve those very basic things. When we look back we'll see we were able to come together and solve our problems, care for one another, build an economy that works for everyone ...'

The optimism is thrilling, a consensus emerging that we had paradise before, in our ordinary lives, and we didn't even know it. But maybe I feel that more intensely anyway since I was certain I was about to die.

One morning in mid-March my nose begins to bleed out of nowhere, drip-drip-dripping straight into my bowl of porridge. *No one needs that of a morning.* It's just one more side effect, nothing to worry about, even though I'm convinced at the time I'm having a prolonged and fatal brain haemorrhage.

Schools begin to close across the UK. More philosophers turn up. 'Humans aren't the problem,' offers one boffin on TV, 'it's our systems. We don't need to vanish to heal the Earth, we need a revolution of policy and ideology that changes the way we interact with the Earth. The problem is our methods, not *us*, and to think otherwise veers into ecofascism.' Crikey. Over in rigidly locked-down Italy, levels of nitrogen dioxide pollution fall drastically. Venetians say the canal water hasn't been this clear in sixty years.

A call comes in from the hospital: a check-up echo heart scan scheduled for May is being brought forward to tomorrow and chaperones can no longer accompany chemo patients. Simon's eyes brim. 'You can't be on your own! With the cold cap and everything!'

I'll be on my own from now on.

The virus news is shocking, societies across the planet imploding. Britain is, say the news reports, 'on the same trajectory as Italy'. Nadine Dorries becomes the first MP to be diagnosed with Covid-19 (and one month later will be promoted to Minister of State for Mental Health, Suicide Prevention and Patient Safety). By 17 March in Ireland all the pubs are closed, effectively cancelling Paddy's Day (to some Irish, worse than cancelling Christmas). Mass graves are being speedily dug in Iran.

Monday 23 March and lockdown arrives in the UK, alongside a text from the NHS: 'We have identified that you're at risk of severe illness if you catch coronavirus.' I'm now officially an NHS 'vulnerable' so must shield my barely functioning immune system. A walk in the park now means heavy-breathing joggers spittle-flecking potential death into the back of my neck, so I won't go anywhere beyond the balcony for the next six weeks. We don't have a garden but our one-bedroom flat, our *own home*, has never felt so precious. The *world* is now closed. Paranoia rules. Death talk is everywhere. Listening to *Steve Wright's Sunday Love Songs* one weekend, he plays 'Wind Beneath My Wings'. Girly sap tears seep from my eyes.

The need to work, thankfully, intervenes and I get back to the story of Amy Winehouse who, in this week's balcony-walking episode, has lost her mobile phone in her beehive. That's the spirit!

Dr Bridger rings to say Covid is now directly affecting my treatment plan. The final hardcore Chemo 4 is being cancelled outright – the Big Guns as it's known – now deemed too risky: should sepsis arrive again there won't be an isolated bed for me anywhere in the hospital. (I visualise the scene: lying on a camp bed, on a drip, in the hospital car park, in a diamond-motif nightie.) 'So, we're going to just crack on,' she declares, undaunted as ever. I'm going straight onto the next chemo, a less toxic, weekly version, bringing my whole plan forward three weeks. It will last between nine and twelve weeks, depending on tolerance (with an antibody 'infusion' every three weeks).

I'm determined not to take Ev up on her driving offer; her dad, with dementia, is in a care home in Scotland; she has more than enough on her plate. Instead, I'm walking the four miles there and back to hospital, seeing as the bus is now a killer-germ capsule on wheels.

The 8 a.m. walk is a metropolitan revelation, birdsong loudly chirruping overhead in every treelined street, traffic almost negligible. The few oncoming pedestrians are emphatically, almost comically swerved. Normally, I'd use the walking time to talk on the phone with a friend or family member, but Simon has banned me from talking in the street, lest a stray virus molecule dangling in the air is sucked into my yapping mouth, even beneath a mask.

On the chemo ward, the atmosphere has dramatically changed – it's edgy, speedy, the strain showing in the eyes of the staff above their now permanent surgical masks. A well-spoken gentleman in a wheelchair, agitated about his susceptibility to Covid, is shouting, 'I tick three cancer boxes!' He demands to see a doctor. No doctor is available, they're all deployed throughout the hospital, on wards hastily reconfigured to treat Covid, as is about to happen to this ward. From my next treatment onwards, the chemo unit will be relocated for the first time in its history. All surgery is now cancelled although 'urgent cancer surgery' will be going ahead in a private hospital elsewhere in London (no doubt at horrific expense to the NHS).

The following week the chemo suite has been moved into the recovery room of the ground-floor day treatment centre;

now, chemo patients can avoid hospital corridors on upper floors percolating with deadly virus. No visitors are allowed anywhere in the hospital. I'll now spend one day every week for the next three months, alone, in a hospital buckling under ever-increasing pressure.

Simon walks me to the next treatment, through Crouch End, where queues have formed outside every store – Waitrose, Co-op, Tesco, Boots, Superdrug – spooked-out humans in masks in single file, at least two metres apart.

The day treatment centre is still being reconfigured into a specialist chemo ward, the effort involving everyone I've known so far from my own chemo team and several strangers. People bustle in with boxes and staff take orders amid supply-chain chaos. 'There's no medium gloves, only small or large!' Wooden cabinets are being carted out, equipment on trolleys carted in, technicians in a quandary fiddling with cables and plugs. 'There's not enough space!'

I've brought my own lunch, made by Simon, and send a message to his mum about the highlight of my day being the delicious tuna sandwich and veg rice combo her son made for me that morning, a text which makes me blub because he's not here and can't distract me through the first twenty minutes of the cold cap. I contemplate abandoning it altogether: attempting to preserve my hair seems pitiful now, not only through all this personal palaver but with the horror of the world outside. I stick with it: there's been so much effort already. The food trolley lady, Joan, is now banned from working, she's over seventy and self-isolating, so Sheila, the finance adviser from Macmillan, takes over her duties. A patient has donated posh Belgian biscuits which become the second highlight of the day.

With no Simon, Ronnie O'Sullivan saves me, my snooker hero, appearing on a new podcast by Colin Murray, called *52*, where random questions are picked via playing cards. O'Sullivan talks about how winning doesn't bring you happiness, nor money, nor any material thing; his happiest years were spent living with a mate on a council estate in Liverpool. His life today, as he always says, is about health, running, eating well and friends, family and community. I smile, remembering how so many of the rich, famous and successful have said this to me over the years.

Brad Pitt once said, in a *Rolling Stone* interview with my old *Smash Hits* chum Chris Heath, 'I'm the guy who has everything, right? Well, let me tell you, as the guy who has everything, once you have everything, all you're left with is yourself.'

This might be true (it is true) but on that particular day, watching the NHS staff around me power on through unprecedented stress, it was also true that a pay rise would bring them significantly more happiness than their current 'reward': a hand-clapping Boris Johnson outside No. 10 of a Thursday evening, encouraging the same from the imprisoned public. Even if, on the first night it happens, there's a genuine emotional response, the residents of our block out in pan-pummelling force, while a lone male voice across the estate sings 'You'll Never Walk Alone'. Meanwhile, in a large back garden near Bedford, a ninety-nine-year-old World War II veteran called Tom is contemplating his walking frame and a modest idea for raising funds for the NHS.

Ev is now back in St Albans, restricted from travelling to Scotland, so now insists she'll pick me up from hospital every single week (and sometimes take me there too). It's a two-hour round trip for her, in a Land Rover Discovery so huge that, when I bolt to the back seat – angry red dents in my forehead where the cold cap has been clamped, hair damp and still freezing – we're approximately *three* metres apart (Professor Chris Whitty would approve). She is now a heroic Thunderbird, nicknamed Parker, chauffeur of Lady Penelope's FAB 1 motor, come to my intercity rescue.

At home NHS letters await. An appointment with Doc Bridger must now happen on the phone. A second MRI scan is cancelled.

I see an interview with the newsreader George Alagiah, about living with both coronavirus and cancer. 'In some ways,' he muses to Sophie Raworth, 'I think that those of us living with cancer are stronger because we kind of know what it is like to go into something where the outcomes are uncertain.' I hope he's right: I'll take solace wherever I can.

It's now apparent that I'm deeply fortunate again: if my diagnosis had come three months later, I might well have been offered no treatment whatsoever, never mind surgery, for at least a year. People will die from cancer because of Covid. It could so very easily have been me. I could've been *actually doomed*, after all.

16

THE SPORTING LIFE

*'The world ain't all sunshine and rainbows.
It's a very mean and nasty place and I don't
care how tough you are, it will beat you to
your knees and keep you there permanently
if you let it. You, me or nobody is gonna hit
as hard as life. But it ain't about how hard
you hit. It's about how hard you can get hit
and keep moving forward. How much you
can take and keep moving forward. That's
how winning is done!'*

Rocky Balboa

Sport. Never played any, not properly anyway. Staggering up
and down the right wing of the hockey team at secondary school
doesn't really count, lacking as I was in the requisite aggression,
audacity and skill. I've tried outdoors running and hated it, feet
thwacking onto the ground causing shaky-brain syndrome that
made clouds overhead rush past like a speeded-up storm.

Growing up in Scotland, skiing was encouraged by the school, trips to Aviemore a winter opportunity to piledrive headfirst into a hillock in a blizzard in minus-ten conditions, as you watch one of your skis sail off down a ravine. Unlike me, Ali, Jill and Ev grew up to be excellent skiers, which meant, in our twenties, skiing holidays to the alpine vistas of Europe, but that's not really sport either; that's an opportunity to piledrive headfirst into a vat of peach schnapps and make a berk of yourself with the Brits Abroad Geezers also on a winter's bender (it wasn't just me).

But I am and always have been a *master* spectator. A world-class champion at numerous hours perched on the sofa's edge shouting, 'Oh no!' (Scotland football team) or, 'C'maaaan!' (Olympics/ Paralympics) or, 'Yeesss!' (whoever is beating Novak Djokovic) or (in the case of Ronnie O'Sullivan), 'He can't pot that, can he!?'

For millions of us – *billions* of us – sport is the ultimate release, an alternative reality where everything to do with your own life is temporarily suspended, all your daily anxieties evaporated, all your unresolved problems to be returned to only when the battle is over – be your problems physical, emotional, cultural, political, all of it. Even if I *was* dying, I'm certain, sport would transcend everything.

There are no sports I loathe other than Formula 1 racing, which is as interesting to me as watching CCTV footage of pimped-up go-carts thundering around the M25. Back in the early nineties I was sent to a swanky Formula 1 racing event in Italy with plume-hatted jazz gonk Jay Kay from Jamiroquai (racing enthusiast and owner of a fleet of Ferraris), given free champagne in scorchio Italian sunshine and seated high up in the grandstand awaiting the 'action'. As the cars squealed around and around – nyeee ... nyeeeee ... *nyeeeeeee!* – I fell sound asleep. Asking Jay Kay afterwards what it feels like to drive, as he had done, at 200 mph, he replied with an informationally barren, 'Quick.'

The rest I've loved from girlhood, especially the global tournaments and very markedly, unlike music, increasingly so the older I become. The first indication of this passion ramping up was, perhaps unsurprisingly, the London Olympics 2012. I'd been away during Super Saturday on 4 August, trapped inside a New York hotel room typing jetlagged sentences on atmospheric art-rock glumsters The XX, being constantly texted by Simon and Gilly B over Mo Farah, Jessica Ennis-Hill and Greg Rutherford's forty-eight minutes of golden athletics triumph.

Back home with Simon, we were running for a bus, hoping to make the stop before the bus pulled away. Clambering on, panting, the waiting driver acknowledged our efforts with both a huge grin and her fingertips pressed on her head: the 'M' of the newly famed 'Mobot'. The city was so fevered, the nation transfixed, the achievements on TV so dazzling, we needed to Be There with our fellow Londoners. An online flurry to buy tickets ensued – too sharpish, as it happened: Simon booked tickets for the Paralympics instead. The Paralympics in 2012 was still an unknown quantity, making its Channel 4 TV debut that year, but we were nonetheless going to Be There. Simon, in an act of solidarity, waved his club foot in the air and yelped, 'These are my people!'

It was *spectacular*. A stunning autumn day, sunbeams sweeping through cobalt skies, the army of seventy thousand volunteer helpers in their purple-and-red tops bearing permanent smiles, pointing giant sponge fingers towards thronging Queen Elizabeth Olympic Park. We saw Clare Balding striding along a path and I couldn't have boggled more if it was Queen Elizabeth herself. We saw athletics in the morning, including the blind long jump, saw Ellie Simmonds win her heat in the afternoon, seated in the top row of an Aquatics Centre so hot we were dripping from our chins. We stayed for the evening even without stadium tickets, watching David Weir win his wheelchair race on a giant screen on-site, cheers roaring outwards from the stadium twenty yards away.

Simon blurted, 'This is like the best festival I've ever been to in my life! Because there's no bloody music!' (Twenty years an author of books on Musical Greats, he remains a music apostle, but increasingly festival phobic. The only time he went to Glastonbury, in 2007, the rain was so bad there were punters canoeing through mud.)

I'd lived in London for twenty-six years by then and never known the city so joyful, the population of this vast, often troubled and dangerous metropolis in the greatest mood of its life. London at its best, Britain at its best, humanity at its best.

But my very favourite sport, since I was a kid, the one where I've never had a buddy who cared like I cared, is snooker. And it's snooker, throughout the first three traumatic months of chemotherapy, which saves me, cocooning me in a parallel dimension safe from all worldly harm. Starting with the Masters in January, to all the spring TV tournaments in the modern year-round season (the Shoot Out, Grand Prix, Welsh Open, Players Championship) until April 2020, when the World Championship is Covid-postponed until August. Swizzed again!

Snooker has saved me for ever, providing a hermetically sealed chrysalis of drama and intensity much preferable to the drama and intensity of the real world beyond the intoxicatingly green baize. Through the penniless freelance years of the late nineties, through the death of my mum, through three miscarriages when I just didn't want to think about anything other than who was going to spanner the irksome new reign of Mark 'The Torturer' Selby. And when snooker's not saving me, it's providing sheer sporting thrills, much of it inducing a synapse-sizzling quiver of nerves wondering just how brilliant/psychotic Ronnie 'The Rocket' O'Sullivan will be when he turns up 'amongst the balls' this time.

My dad introduced me to snooker in 1975, when I was ten and he was fifty-four. We'd watch *Pot Black* in the small TV Room mid-house and he'd explain these fascinating, intricate rules; which colour equalled how many points, what 'needing a snooker' meant, about ingenious safety manoeuvres and how all the best players potted at speed. It was the era of Ray 'Dracula' Reardon and Dennis 'Upside-Down Specs' Taylor and I loved it all: the hush of the comperes, the clack of the immaculately shiny balls, the luminous white gloves of the shadowy referees, the silence of the crowd until something astounding happened – either a winner or a howler – causing a synchronised eruption of 'Oooooh!' or a clatter of raucous applause. By 1980, snooker was a UK TV force, a sporting phenomenon engineered by buccaneering sports promotor Barry Hearn (also manager of flame-haired Romford Robot, Steve 'Interesting' Davis). We watched the world finals together for *hours*, when the most important thing happening on Earth in May 1980 was whether me 'n' dad's hero, Alex 'Hurricane' Higgins, could bedazzle once more and see off Cliff 'The Grinder' Thorburn (disaster, he couldn't). Then, in the '82 finals, Higgins beat Reardon – 'Yesssss!' – the final all fans remember for the tearful beckoning of Higgins to his wife and baby daughter. My dad's beguiling, Egyptian-almond eyes filled with tears that night and I didn't really understand why. I was seventeen years old, a chaotic post-punk music obsessive, fond of the booze and fags – much like my mother, a woman I know my dad loved dearly but who had plummeted since the mid-seventies into the alcoholism he was powerless to do anything about. She often worked night shifts but on the evenings she didn't they'd drink, behind the fully closed door of The Front Room (the proper lounge), my dad matching her drink for drink, saying the share of Famous Grouse whisky he drank was 'a half she won't get' (he could cope with it, where she couldn't).

Maybe, I used to think, because of his war experience, Dad could cope with anything. In Burma, he'd been one of those malnourished, abused and forgotten men of the Second World War who built the Thailand to Burma railway, immortalised in the movie *The Bridge on the River Kwai*. For three and a half years he'd seen unspeakable things that he barely mentioned, other than grisly descriptions of the maggots in the rice at the bottom of his mess tin, the food his cell mate told him he must eat, 'because it's your passport back to Blighty'. He told us, though, about the fate of his cell mate, a Dutchman, who was murdered by a Japanese soldier, shot in the head for no reason, in front of my dad's eyes, the two men having taught each other their native languages to keep their minds alive. Back in Scotland, blind from myriad wartime diseases and close to death, he was nursed back to life by my mum, a newly qualified nurse, and was able to walk, laugh, eat and see again. He always said, when he couldn't see, he fell in love with her voice first. In 1947 they were married and their bond, no matter what, for forty-two years until his death, was unbreakable.

He was, in some ways, an enigma to me. Born in 1919 he was almost Edwardian, his life experience unimaginable. Perhaps this made me love him all the more, a truly gentle man, kind, enthusiastic and protective, funny on the quiet, who'd lose himself playing piano, beautifully, on an antique wooden upright. He loved the absurdism of Spike Milligan, the raucous country music of Johnny Cash and when we watched our beloved snooker, I saw a look on his face of both delighted pleasure and relief. I think snooker, for him, was exactly what it became for me: a refuge, an escape, as comforting a psychic insulation as heroin (I'd imagine). It's also just like every other sport: tense, exhilarating, featuring your personally appointed goodies and baddies, a duel between good and evil.

In 1989, Dad lay dying. I held his hand on his deathbed, my fingers wrapped around his slender piano fingers, hooked up to a morphine drip, not so different to the drip on the pole with the castors I'd come to know so well thirty years into the future. I traced a finger around the hospital wristband spelling out his name and date of birth.

'Nineteen-nineteen,' I said out loud. 'That was a long time ago.'

He smiled, eyes closing, drifting into the rainbow colours of the morphine dream-state and oblivion beyond.

I watched snooker alone from then on, witnessing throughout the nineties the domination of our sport, our bonding bedrock, by the clinically ruthless boy-machine Stephen Hendry.

'Best off out of it, Dad!' I'd shout to the sky, with a smile, knowing how much he would've disapproved of Hendry and loved Ronnie O'Sullivan instead. The Rocket detonated into the sport in 1992, by '95 a nineteen-year-old Masters winner, a wayward, brilliant, belligerent force of nature as befitting to the snooker year of 1995 as Liam Gallagher was in the crucible of rock'n'roll.

In 2012, the Masters tournament moved from Wembley Arena to Alexandra Palace, a ten-minute walk across Alexandra Park from our flat, and two years later the finally hooked Simon (I had a snooker buddy at last) bought us tickets to see Ronnie play in the quarter finals (sixteen pounds – a snip!).

Ronnie strolled into the intimate, curtained-off area deep inside the Palace, all dressed in black, raven hair glistening, the Elvis of snooker and I gasped out loud, 'I can't believe he's real!' (Even though I'd been interviewing famous people for decades.) He was playing Ricky 'So Boring He Doesn't Even Have a Nickname' Walden and in a devastating virtuoso performance whitewashed him 6–0 in fifty-eight rocketing minutes.

In 2018 we saw Ronnie again at the Masters, in the first round, playing Marco 'Full of Eastern Promise' Fu and what followed was a Ronnie performance so exquisite, so deadly, so unfathomably, effortlessly accurate it entered the realm of the absurd. By the mid-session interval Ronnie was not only 4–0 up via three centuries, but Fu hadn't even been given the *chance* to pot a single ball. Walking out for a quick pint during the interval, a bloke behind us boggled to his buddy, 'This is gettin' silly now!' Ronnie returned and carried on for a 6–0 whitewash in a match where the most memorable moment for Fu, a former world No. 5, was a fly landing, pointedly, on his forehead.

In January 2022 we saw Ronnie at The Masters *again* – the first crowd event we'd been to since 2019, by now triple Covid-vaccinated and willing to take an audience-based risk. After 2021's Masters had been staged behind closed doors, the noise as Ronnie strode into the arena was electrifying, the Ally Pally fans more vocal than any I'd ever known in forty-five years of engagement with this traditionally sedate spectator sport; a crowd who'd not only missed *a* crowd, but *this* crowd, of snooker fans just like them. On their way to the commentary box Steve Davis and Stephen Hendry waved to the crowd, my eighties' and nineties' nemeses, both commentary giants today, especially Hendry, whose brilliant analysis, both psychological and technical, is the most mercilessly insightful in the history of the game (even you, Dad, would appreciate him now).

Ronnie shimmered once more, dressed in his signature black, his movement around the table somewhere between a prowl and a dance, like a waltzing panther, now the most successful snooker player in history and newly psychologically serene. He beat the charismatic, talented and underachieving Jack 'Jackpot' Lisowski 6–1, so gracious in defeat he noted the walk-on cheer for his opponent and childhood hero was, 'the loudest roar from a crowd I've ever heard'. After these unique two years of global incarceration – exactly two years for me of often-grim physical trauma – the simultaneous exhilaration of this sporting moment and the ongoing road to wellness was no less than elevational, lifting me off my seat, thrilled, hollering, the universe whole again.

And four months later, when he finally equalled Stephen Hendry's seven world titles at the Crucible in Sheffield with yet another peerless masterclass, I sat on the sofa and wept and wept, even more than Ronnie did himself that night, draped over the shoulders of his opponent Judd 'The Ace In The Pack'

Trump, uncontrollably sobbing, for several long minutes. This was, unquestionably, one of the greatest and most emotionally affecting moments in sporting history. Simon told me I cried more openly at Ronnie's win, 'actual *heaving*' – with relief, jubilation, a sense of justice, this culmination of a twenty-year wait – than I did when I was told I didn't have terminal cancer. Hendry said it was 'an honour' to share the seven-title achievement with British sport's most under-celebrated genius, 'because he's taken the game to another level. He plays the game the way it's supposed to be played. He is an artist.'

> An artist, in my eyes, is someone who can lighten up a dark room. I have never and will never find difference between the pass from Pelé to Carlos Alberto in the final of the World Cup in 1970, and the poetry of the young Rimbaud – Eric Cantona[1]

The passion that flames within every sporting fanatic can, at times, block out rationality and once, in my case, the configuration of my Scottish DNA. Then again, perhaps it was the fault of a *different* kind of passion.

During the 2002 World Cup, I was consumed by a flagrant crush on David Beckham, as was much of the planet, the newly anointed England captain leading his boys into battle in Japan. This meant, for the first time in history, I was cheering on an England football team (not that I took much notice of the rest of the England team).

I loved David Beckham. I loved David Beckham, originally, because of his talent (it's *absolutely true*), since he scored that goal from the halfway line against Wimbledon in 1996, as audaciously rock'n'roll a manoeuvre as anyone had pulled off in the whole of the Britpop era. Through the late 1990s, the sarong-wearing pioneer of the 'metrosexual' became more culturally luminous by the day, a dazzling, constant distraction for me through personally dismal years, including London-renting calamities where I was forced to move nine times in eighteen months.

By 2001 David Beckham was less a football player, more an emblem of still-burgeoning Celebrity Culture itself, a multi-platform brand, a multimillionaire, a fiercely debated style icon and as famous as anyone had ever been. His beauty, coupled with his gift and his mesmerising demeanour – this curiously zen-state dreaminess which promised so much sexual allure – conspired in me to see less a human being, more an actual Angel of Light who glowed from within.

In 2001, I even spent a few hours in his company, interviewing him for *The Face* magazine, the first sportsperson ever to appear on the cover, which was, he beamed, 'an 'onna [an honour]'. I also witnessed his no doubt fragrant underpants during a change of clothes at the photoshoot, whisking his jeans off in front of me and just standing there, for ages, and I'm sorry (no I'm not) but you would just stare, wouldn't you, *really rather a lot?* He saw me staring at his crotch and looked across with The Beckham Smile, the one which explodes like a flashbulb to this day, and my knees turned to Cadbury's Caramel.

Ali, of course, loathed David Beckham, being a Scotswoman who would rather set fire to her own head than support anything to do with the England football team. That year, she and her Irish husband, Billy, invited me on holiday to his family hometown, Rosslare, where I could stay in the cosy family caravan in his folks' garden. We watched all the World Cup matches, which involved morning drinking, seeing as they were happening in the Far East, a lethal combination which, come the quarter finals against Brazil, saw me shouting for England (when I really meant Beckham), surrounded by Guinness-quaffing Irishmen in a boozer at 10 a.m., all wearing the shirts of any country as long as it wasn't England. Ali was appalled. 'Just you get back to yer caravan!' she bawled, as we wobbled away from the pub, 'I've had enough of you and yer

Beckham shite!' And so I spent the rest of the day in the caravan, the dog house, in disgrace, on my football holidays that summer of 2002. Oh, how we can laugh about it now.

Back in 1998, I had a conversation with Nicky Wire, the Manic Street Preachers' effervescent, feather boa-tossing bass player, which has stayed with me ever since. Then twenty-nine, he'd already lost his manager to cancer and his best friend, the Manic's talisman Richey Edwards, to presumed suicide aged just twenty-seven.

'There's two things I couldn't live without and that's sport and chips,' announced the luminous rock star, with his fabled dazzling grin. 'If there was a choice between music and never seeing the Olympics again or Wales play rugby again, I'd [comedy thumb out to the left] *ditch music.*'

Back then I kind of knew what he meant, but now I definitely know. The Paralympics 2012, all those Ronnies at the Masters: days I wouldn't have swapped for a decade of Glastonbury Festivals.

Like so many aspects of our lives during the global pandemic, it was only when sport was taken away that we appreciated how much we needed it. Sport is so much more than entertainment (essential enough in itself); it's DNA-deep, wrapped up in your actual belief system, your sense of community and belonging. Your team, and your individual heroes, are ultimately projections of yourself, which is why it hurts so much when they lose. Because *you* lose, too. Back in the nineties, I had a flatmate I dubbed 'Football Shaun', a footie fanatic who loved sport so much he was manager of a Ladbrokes betting emporium, whose team was (unfeasibly, for a northerner) Chelsea. Whenever Chelsea lost he was unable to speak, literally, for up to three consecutive days. But this level of devotion is worth it, always, because our sporting heroes' wins, equally, are our wins, a shared history, a shared *story*, of struggle and achievement, through generations of spectacular human drama, an eternal lifeline of hope in the often-wretched unfairness of everyday reality.

Sport is truly a different dimension: sport is rules, structure and logic, it's work equals achievement, it's the power of the mind (often much more than the body), it's a superhuman skillset the majority of us can never attain and an ancient global culture where opinion, ultimately, doesn't matter. Sport is *actually* fair, it's clear winners and losers, it's numbers, equations and infinitesimal margins, it's rare empirical certainty. In a world which certainly ain't all sunshine and rainbows, which can be viciously mean and nasty, it's as far away from the worst of reality as it's possible to go. And, in snooker especially, it's given me one of the longest, most reliable and most life-affirming relationships of my life.

So, thanks, Dad, for giving me, your now fifty-seven-year-old youngest daughter (who is not so wayward any more), something which lasts for ever, which has saved me, time and time and time and time again. Which is maybe the very definition of what a Proper Dad does. He also gave me something else which has saved me for decades: the opportunity to own my own home.

17

HOMEWARD BOUND

It's been seventeen years now since I was able to buy my own flat, something I could never have done without inheriting thirty-two thousand pounds from my parents' estate after the death of my mum in 2004. My dad, an insurance accountant, who loathed being an insurance accountant, had made sure my mum would be financially stable after his death, knowing she would be anything but stable otherwise; a vulnerable, lonely woman with few friends, still possessed by what she always called the 'demon alcohol'. Leaving their final home together in the isolated countryside, she moved into her own three-bedroom semi on the outskirts of Perth where she lived until her death, the proceeds of the property then split between myself and my three remaining siblings (we'd lost Ronnie back in '87 to a pulmonary embolism, at the age my mum always spelled out as 'Thirty-seven and a half').

In 2005, I sat in a financial adviser's office, a hitherto alien environment, and was told I could afford a place of my own for £120,000. Months followed of being told by several nettle-faced estate agents, 'You'll never find any kind of flat in London for that money.' Months later still I found one for exactly that money, mainly because it belonged to an elderly couple, with décor unchanged from the 1970s. It wasn't even merely a studio, it was a proper, one-bedroom, second-floor flat in a block in Hornsey, north London, and today you couldn't buy a refurbished bike hangar on a London car-parking space for that money.

Moving-in date was 7 October 2005, excitedly turning the key into an empty shell which needed the full refurbishment of every room, costing every carrot I had left (post-deposit and solicitors' fees). After two decades of turbulent London renting, this remains the most sensible and life-enhancing decision I have ever made.

It's primal, of course. A sense of safety, stability, security and autonomy – a foundational layer of Maslow's 'hierarchy of needs' – which becomes ever more vital the moment serious illness brings into your life extra levels of fear and vulnerability. Coupled with the lockdown shock of 2020, the preciousness of my own home had never been more pronounced. With this newly heightened appreciation, thoughts also turned to the plight of those for whom home means something else: physical danger, emotional suffocation or the daily miseries of a leaky, damp, substandard space from which there is no escape. The opposite, in fact, of what home is supposed to mean or certainly means to me: a sanctuary, safe from harm.

Back in the 1980s, when I believed in The Revolution, when I believed in the 'property is theft' dictum (one borrowed from the French, *naturellement*), vowing never to capitulate to the capitalist lie of 'mortgages, fridges and pensions', I had no idea what I was talking about. I was a foaming, power-to-the-people idealist for whom people who owned stuff were The Enemy and we paupers who had nothing were The Noble Oppressed. Same old girl? I'm not that girl, any more. At least, not in the twenty-first century. One day humanity might actually evolve out of capitalism, man, which serves only the needs of the market, into the utopia of global fairness. On such a planet all our resources would be shared, each human being with a decent, safe place to live, with access to clean water, plenty of sustainable food, affordable energy from the infinite elements and no deluded psychos dropping bombs on blameless heads. For now, though, a home of my own (alongside the person who shares it with me) is the central ballast of my life.

In 2020, though, because we're always at home through both cancer and Covid, there's no escaping the deterioration, as there would be after years of no meaningful upkeep. We've had a leaky roof for years – a roof owned by the council, who take months to repair anything and, even when they do, the problems always resurface. During heavy rain, water either drip-drip-drips or *cascades* through the slim, horizontal ventilation shafts serving our kitchen and bedroom windows, loosening and blackening wallpaper, damaging the already corroded and paint-chipped wooden window-sill seats. Leaks elsewhere cause water damage in the hallway and a corner of the living room. Simon, hitherto the least practical man in Britain (living with the least practical woman), uses his considerable creative skills to at least alleviate the window leaks. Sheets of tinfoil are patchworked together with gaffer tape, taped underneath the ventilation shafts and fashioned to form a sluice, tapering towards small, secondary, top windows. He then hangs the sluice through permanently open windows: just the ticket for the rains of chilly winter.

The kitchen is falling apart. It was all I could afford at the time, a basic, one-wall galley from Ikea. Today, two supposedly 'country cottage effect' parallel wooden shelves are drooping at dangerous angles, caked in grime, underneath which is a bolted-on, basic steel pole for the dangling of cooking implements. The effect is less country cottage, more 'found some stuff in a skip and drilled it into the wall', a highly flawed, overly romantic idea where proper wall cupboards should always have been. Crockery and sundry utensils are crammed into either one stand-alone cupboard on the floor or the old-school pantry in the corner, which is stuffed with not only all the essential, non-perishable foods but the iron, Tupperware bowls, storage jars, tea-lights, plastic bags, tote bags, blankets and admin boxes from fifteen years ago.

The overhead lighting appears even more unseemly when it's switched on, all the better to see the three-way spotlight ceiling plate encrusted in years of upwardly wafting cooking grease. Directly above the cooker, these upward wafts have also left a large, oily ceiling stain. The worktop, made from half-price real wood – which, again, I thought romantic – has decayed around the sink, especially at the back; deep, black pockets of rot now home at night to shoals of darting silverfish, the result of never sealing the worktop as you're supposed to. Above the worktop are rows of orange-and-white chequered tiles, painted by me back in 2006 to mask the 1950s' floral design below, now ruined, with peeling paint, irredeemably discoloured grouting and chipped around the edges.

The washing machine malfunctions; it can't fill itself up from the mains pipe (the high-street store fitter insisted the water pressure was too low and left us to it), so for years we've attached a bendy hose to the sink tap, laboriously filling the machine by hand. An ill-fitting DIY effort, the hose routinely pings off from the gushing cold tap and floods the already rotting worktop. Our kitchen table has always been too big, hinderingly big, taking up a third of the room, a lovely table, yes, a coppery-orange expanse of slat-effect wood with that supposed country-ish feel (and a circular burn mark from a tea-light, the result of coaster-free life). It was chosen by me in an industrial estate showroom without measuring, convinced it was the kind of table, in the most misguidedly romantic delusion of them all, you'd see in the paintings of Vincent van Gogh.

Beneath the mammoth table is a towering tenement of cardboard boxes housing further historical admin alongside sentimental trinkets and gifts I cannot bear, yet cannot bear to throw away. Sporadically, I've emptied these boxes out (only to fill them up again), a manoeuvre involving a box-shunting shock to the cosy tenement dwellers, a speedy platoon of spiders then unleashed across the kitchen floor, as if a spider's-own version of the British army were going 'over the top' in the First World War.

The doors of the cupboard under the sink, where blackened pots reside in a grey plastic laundry basket, are now hanging at jaunty angles, paint peeling off, while the open gaps between the sink unit, washing machine, cooker and fridge are not big enough for any human arm to reach through with a disinfectant cloth. The gaps, therefore, have housed years of toppling foodstuffs, creating multi-layered archaeological digs on the also-rotting wooden floorboards, a handy haven for those spiders on the run from their demolished cardboard tenement on the other side of the room.

Simon is the chef, a fantastic cook, who spends much of his life in this room attempting to keep us nourished, especially in these calamitous times, both incarcerated and illness compromised. One day, he walks into the kitchen and looks palpably forlorn.

'I love the flat, you know I still love the flat but ... this makes me feel depressed,' he says, surveying the tinfoil sheets, the grimy shelves and the gaps to the spider's graveyard. 'It's ... Sad Kitchen.'

He's right. I've known it for years. His words are unbearable, I feel like I've failed him, after all his efforts to keep me alive through the most physically feeble year of my life, all the creative joy he brings to cooking and he can't even do it in a civilised space. We have a roof over our heads, yes – albeit a leaky one – but we're living on the edge of bum-life. I'm beyond embarrassed. *Ashamed.* Surely I can change things. I *must*.

In autumn of 2020 a windfall comes my way, suddenly and very unexpectedly paid a fee I was owed from some years ago (an occasional freelance hazard). Stunned and thrilled, I squirrel the money away, thinking it might form the basis, one day, of the funds for a new kitchen.

Like many of us, if lockdown provided one positive outcome, it was the money we saved from being imprisoned at home.

Restrictions aside, for half of 2020 I wasn't even drinking, because I couldn't, or eating much, because I couldn't, used zero public transport, had negligible nights out, went on no holidays and spent no disposable income on anything other than an occasional flat white coffee from the only open emporiums on the ghostly local high streets. So maybe I *could* afford a new kitchen, soon. Though it would be months, still, before any workmen – or any other humans – would be allowed through the front door. Until the Covid vaccines still in development, in fact, were finally publicly available.

And until I'd negotiated many more months of 'the process' of treatment, including that time I was convinced I was about to die on the bathroom floor.

18

APRIL FOOL

It's Italy-level hot in London in April 2020 and I'm freezing – cellular-level chilled – wandering up and down the sun-baked balcony with three layers on, including the bobbly woollen jumper with the look and weight of a Himalayan yeti. The mouth is disintegrating, again, sores along the inside of the lips, the side of the tongue, blood vessels bursting in star shapes on the roof of my mouth. Even tongue resting on teeth hurts, while a swig of fizzy water stings, badly. After a call to the chemo unit I'm prescribed codeine which doesn't help. Only Difflam mouthwash every half-hour does, the anti-inflammatory, painkilling gargle which makes having a mouth tolerable.

Eating is now a serious problem and Simon, as ever, wants to help, makes me cold gazpacho soup. It's both delicious and torturous to get through, sip by tiny sip, burning onto lips and tongue like a bowl of pureed Scotch bonnets. Determined to finish it, I take paracetamol, wait thirty minutes, and try again. No improvement, even when each spoonful is positioned directly into the back of the throat. I google what it's possible to eat with this ruinous condition (the grimly titled 'mucositis', a common side effect of chemo) and discover vital information: the main foods to avoid are 'onion, garlic and acidic food like tomatoes'. Bullseye!

Milky-white cheek sores are soon moving backwards into my throat, even the dangly bit at the back – who knew it was called the 'uvula'? – one large, white sore clinging to the side, like lagging. Meals for the day are one tiny Alpro coconut yoghurt, a few spoons of cottage cheese, a small mound of egg mayonnaise and a nectarine whizzed to the mush of baby food, which still hurts, because natural sugars are painful. Even a few sips of unsweetened soya milk sting.

At first, I'm not worried. At five-foot six-and-a-half-inches, I'm a hearty ten stone; I can lose a stone and stay normal. A stone falls off in two weeks. Then another half a stone. This kind of plummeting weight loss is never a good look. All you look like is someone who has cancer. A sick person. A dying person. With caved-in cheeks, shoulder bones visibly poking upwards through skin and oddly muscle-free limbs. Slim people who are healthy do not look like this. Simon calls me Boney P, in 'tribute' to German disco-funk titans Boney M. And now, the annual sporting tournament I look forward to most, the World Snooker Finals in late April, is postponed, my only respite watching the worldwide hit documentary *Tiger King*, on Netflix, an hour peering through a porthole into someone else's madness.

I dread the moment of waking up, which usually happens at 4 a.m., when I immediately begin to silently weep. The first waking sensation is a stab in the back of the throat, as if with a scalpel, made worse on attempts to swallow. Then the stinging fires up, everywhere, an invasion of furious wasps. My pillow is drenched in drool.

Drool. I'm actually drooling. I might as well be 109!

Tracks of dried drool snake across my cheek. And I'd wondered, before all this started, why it was that sex, we always hear, is the last thing on a cancer patient's mind.

Easter Monday and the dangly bit at the back of the throat is now fully swathed in a silky white coat of fungal infection. More flecks of soreness have reached the throat wall. That's enough now. I phone the chemo unit emergency number, who recommend I come in quickly, to ambulatory care, the cab customised with a Perspex Covid barrier screen between driver and passenger. 'Bloods' are taken, neutrophil count 1.7, the low end of normal. At least I don't have sepsis. A doctor takes swabs of the back of my throat, like a throat scrape with steel wool. There's nothing they can do until a long-scheduled check-up appointment with The Doc tomorrow. 'Keep taking codeine' is the only advice; when I do I feel like I always do on painkillers, like I'm living underwater, wading every day through a dense, slow-moving undertow.

It's been two weeks of torture, which has felt like ten months, when I walk into The Doc's consulting room – and succumb to pink-faced tears. She reaches, silently, wearing her mask, for the box of tissues permanently housed on her desk. Pressing one to my bloodshot, sleepless eyes, I let it all hang out.

'I'm sorry! I've just waited so long to see you.'

'Don't worry, let me see.' She shines a torch inside my mouth, down my throat. 'It's particularly nasty,' she concludes. 'Have you had herpes before?'

'Herpes? No!'

'You might have had it and not known and the chemo has brought it out. Well, this is something you're particularly susceptible to. Do you smoke?'

She's forgotten I've already told her.

'I had a vape until January which I've given up. No real cigarettes for many years.'

'OK.'

Oh God, she knows all about the damage done. All those toxic fumes passing through the membrane for all those decades. No wonder it's weak. Smoking might not have given me cancer, but it's given me a big cancer treatment problem. My fault, my fault – all my fault.

Prescriptions follow: more Difflam, anti-fungal pills, herpes pills, twelve bottles of Ensure Plus (a fortified anti-malnutrition milkshake) and a substantial bottle of liquid morphine. She changes my treatment plan again, reduces the dose of the weekly chemo and cancels the session due the following week, allowing me a chance to recover. When I pick the medications up from my local chemist, he nods at the large morphine bottle: 'Keep that in your bag, so no one sees it!' Imagine: being robbed and possibly stabbed and killed on the streets of London for your cancer medication.

The last time I took morphine was recreationally, back in the 1990s, when I was having a brief romantic dalliance with a young man known as Essex, because he looked like twinkle-eyed seventies' pop gypsy David Essex. He took me to see his local football team, Portsmouth FC, where his favourite tipple materialised from a rucksack. A bottle of morphine. Which I also swigged from, despite knowing nothing about morphine. I watched no footie action, swooning instead at the hypnotic 'morphing' of the dreamy cloud formations overhead. This time, all the morphine does is make me slump onto my desk during the day, woozy and foggy, eyelids involuntarily closing. It's also stopping me Going To The Bathroom.

I've been an enthusiastic morning tea-drinker for ever, many piping-hot brews, delicious and satisfying, and now have a new breakfast tea routine: teabag in bottom of mug, one-third hot water, big swirl to make sure I release some caffeine, large helping of unsweetened soya milk, larger helping of tap water from bottled water in the fridge. It's the only way I can tolerate even a few swigs of tepid swill.

I didn't know it was possible to miss a nice cup of tea this much.

The good old days were only three months ago, when life's greatest pleasure was food, wandering Sainsbury's contemplating online-recommended, immune system-boosting superfoods – pomegranates in salads and turmeric-tasty soups. Now, I'm drinking cold tea and sipping from a plastic bottle of anti-malnutrition vanilla milkshake, through a straw. Forming words is such tongue-battering agony I stop talking altogether. Work on the Amy book, until I can speak again, is paused.

The Fear erupts: what if chemo is cancelled outright because I simply can't tolerate it? I'm treatable, all I want is to be treated, but the treatment is killing me. I fantasise about being put into an induced coma for months, so they can still give me treatment and feed me through a drip. I think about those among us in pain every day, the millions who live with chronic pain and I understand why they begin to give up. I beseech the world in my head.

People of the world: rejoice every day you can eat! Rejoice every day you are not in pain! Rejoice every day you can taste and swallow and nourish your body and mind, for you are truly in paradise!

Twentieth of April. Adolf Hitler's birthday. I've been taking morphine for a week, the mouth incrementally improving. Words, tentatively, can form again. I'm well enough for a walk, on another beautiful spring day, marvelling at the candelabras in fulsome bloom on dozens of horse chestnut trees which circle the park.

Simultaneously, I haven't Been To The Bathroom for several days. I'd heard this might happen with morphine (to a lesser degree with codeine) but until now I'd been OK. Back home I take a sachet of Laxido laxative from a small stash I have on standby. An hour later, I really need to Go To The Bathroom. And can't. At all. Severe constipation, like I've never known before. Seated on the loo I'm sweating, loudly straining; this is incredibly painful and increasingly frightening. Nothing budges. I take another Laxido.

Over the next two hours a blockage begins building and building up inside my bowel. I can not only feel it within I can feel it *outwith*. Placing a hand beneath my backside, the whole area is now distended, skin bulging outwards, a huge mass wedged up against my anus, which is as tightly closed as the cork in a bottle of forty-year-old Beaujolais. I start to panic, I must expel this thing and don't know how to – other than to sit on the loo straining, then crying and straining, ever more loudly, the sound of childbirth bursting from my scarlet, vein-popping face. I've flashbacks of the horrifying documentary about Whitney Houston, when her drug-addicted life induced a similar scenario and Bobby Brown attempted to help his wife by digging his fingers into her anus to dislodge the offending mass. Simon, who can hear everything, is now shouting through the bathroom door, offering to do the same.

I DON'T THINK SO.

Shocked, repelled, mortified, I can only attempt to do the same myself – poke, poke, poke, the horror! – but still this thing won't move. I'm now frightened for my *life*, certain my bowel is about to tear open and I'll die on the bathroom floor, knickers at my ankles, distended ass full of sewage, making the death of Elvis Presley seem serene and dignified by comparison.

I'm frenzied, need professional help, ring the Northern pharmacy in tears. A calm woman tells me I now need suppositories and many more laxative sachets, but of course I cannot walk. Simon sprints to the local chemist, as best he can, on his wonky legs, a flailing vision giving Paralympian champ Richard Whitehead a run for his money while I lie face down on our bed. Now, I'm having flashbacks to my childhood home, where the dog of our elderly next-door neighbour wandered its jungly garden with a large pancake of dogshit tragically and possibly fatally stuck to its backside.

Simon sprints back and, still on the bed, I try the suppository. 'Funnily' enough I can't insert it. There's no room to insert it, is there? I'm howling, certain something is about to rupture, ring the chemo unit again, who put me through to ambulatory care. Because of Covid, they can't risk anyone coming into hospital unless it's a top priority emergency so they're sending an ambulance with enema equipment. I'm back on the loo, straining and straining and straining ... *Nothing.*

Simon is now so traumatised by the noise he's wearing earplugs, blocking out at least some of this endless torpor. Lying face down on the bed again I pass out for an hour. On waking up, I put my hand underneath my backside and the bulk is no longer there.

Where the hell's it all gone then!?

The mass, somehow, has been sucked back in. I can now use a suppository!

Twenty minutes later I hear a squeak from deep within my bowel, park on the toilet and wait, terrified, convinced the rupture is on its way. A piercing shriek projectiles from my mouth as an enormous object plummets at speed out of my backside, so large it causes a splashback, the relief as gigantic as it is instant.

Oh dear God, it's out. THANK GOD IT'S OUT. I wonder what it looks like. What could something like that possibly look like!?

The pan is milky, I can't see clearly, so I plunge my hand in and scoop it out. It's like a meteorite made of individual rocks all collided together as one, to form a squat, Mr Whippy-ice-cream-shaped boulder. It's significantly bigger than my fully outstretched hand, wider and taller. To have this thing released from my body took five and a half hours. Even given the mouth-and-throat hell of the last few weeks – beyond anything to do with enduring cancer – this has been one of the very worst things that's ever happened to me. And just when I thought, I say wryly to Simon, that things couldn't get any worse. Which reminds me of a phrase I once heard from irksome nineties' nemesis Damon Albarn, around the year 2000. 'You never know what's round the corner,' he smiled, knowingly, 'but don't get too excited, 'cos you never know what's round the corner ...'

The ambulatory care enema is cancelled. It's Monday night and the *University Challenge* final is on. I watch, have an evening meal of two sips of unsweetened soya milk and go to bed.

When I next see The Doc she is horrified: she forgot to tell me I must regularly take laxatives alongside this level of morphine. She apologises. By that time, because I've been taking codeine instead, I have a thirty-sachet, family-sized box of Laxido ready in my bathroom cabinet. And plentiful suppositories.

I don't touch the morphine ever again.

19

PARK LIFE

Ally Pally means ... 196 acres of nature ... dancing on ice ... a Grade II listed fixer-upper ... London's largest independent music venue ... darts, daredevils and fireworks ... a pint with a view ... London's oldest new theatre ... young Londoners finding their voices ... so much to so many of us. Help us keep it alive and well. Search "Ally Pally Support" to find out how. THANK YOU.

So bugles the tarpaulin billboard affixed to a fence at the top of Alexandra Park, an advert celebrating what's become one of London's best-known landmarks, Alexandra Palace and Park. Our flat sits on an edge of this stunning stretch, a haven for dog-walkers, joggers, picnickers and strolling lovers, where thickets, woods and meadows are lovingly and expertly maintained.

At the park's summit sits Alexandra Palace, the 'People's Palace', which opened on 24 May 1873 and famously burned down sixteen days later (only the outer walls survived), was speedily rebuilt and reopened in May 1875. In 1900 it became a charitable trust, the trustees' duty to keep both building and park 'available for the free use and recreation of the public forever'. The building's vast stone structure holds the history of not only London but Britain; it was used as a refugee camp for displaced Belgians in the First World War, then an internment camp for German and Austrian citizens, became the site of the first BBC broadcast in 1936, survived Doodlebug bomb damage through the Second World War (including the blowing out of the front-central rose window) and in 1980 suffered a second blaze ignited beneath the organ, which destroyed half the building. Rebuilt once more, an ice rink was installed in 1990 (home of rehearsals today for ITV's *Dancing On Ice*) and in 2018 its original 1875 theatre was refurbished and reopened via Lottery Heritage funds.

Affectionately known as Ally Pally, it hosts not only the World Snooker Masters but the PDC World Darts Championship, as well as numerous fayres and festivals and a full spectrum of live music events. There's also a large pub, a boating lake and café, a nine-hole pitch-and-putt golf club, a cricket, rugby and football field, a skateboard park and a Go Ape! climbing walkway.

Ally Pally and Park has it all and has seen it all. And it's known to myself and Simon, simply, as Our Garden. Without which, during 2020/21, we would've comprehensively lost our minds.

London, like all the best major cities, is unexpectedly green; it's almost a secret, a magical aspect of the capital which enhances the lives of millions. Right now, as I type, there's a crow on a wire through the kitchen window, the same wire a demented squirrel is often seen darting along, upside down. A glade of wooded greenery beyond the wire is home to the foxes we regularly see bolting behind cars near rubbish bins or (just once) audaciously sashaying down the middle of the road with a large, triangular slice of pizza hanging from its teeth. It's 9.30 a.m. and there's still frost on the ground; big, healthy brown rats scramble into bushes, the bare winter branches and twigs of the horse chestnut tree directly in front of the window betray a magpie's sometime nest at its heart, currently being refurbished by an enterprising squirrel (maybe even the upside-down squirrel). This tree, our tree, has brought the changing of the seasons directly into our living space every year for the last seventeen – the eternal cycle of birth, bloom, decay, death and regeneration just one reason I've no desire to live in a primarily hot country.

When I was a youngster, I didn't see any of this. Not *really* see it – as in, acknowledge it, appreciate it, love it. Even as The Four of Us were rolling around Perth's Inches, home not only to towering trees but to watery wildlife, we paid no attention to any of it, too busily obsessed with boys and music and clothes and more boys and who was up for *Grease* at the pictures, *again?* Today, all these decades later, especially through the sensory deprivations of both lockdown and illness (no alcohol, nicotine, delicious food, hot cups of tea, right good kiss-ups or cavorting through life with chums), the natural world outside this window provides all the oxygen, pleasure and inspiration I need to survive.

After six full weeks of not walking further than the balcony around our block (other than the day trip to chemotherapy), I gingerly set forth parkwards, avoiding paths, across the grassland towards Ally Pally where, standing underneath the iconic rose window looking south, every one of the London skyline characters stand proud in the recognition line-up. Most of them didn't exist when I moved to London in 1986: to the east, a landed space ship that would dwarf Bell's Sports Centre, the impressive new Tottenham Hotspur football stadium, alongside the monolithic giants of the City (known to me as The Towers of Bastards), along towards the Gherkin, the Walkie-Talkie, the Shard, the Cheesegrater, St Paul's Cathedral to the west and the BT tower, for ever known to us kids-of-the-seventies as the one the kitten pushes over in the 'Kitten Kong' episode of *The Goodies*. But up here all of that, below, is someone else's dream. Up here is where the magpies bounce, the crows squawk and the seagulls sit, legless on the grass, nature's dreamscape knolls and meadows and woods painting themselves, so cleverly, in the colours and shades and textures of every season and every increment in between. Through the pandemic I must've walked around this park a thousand times, never bored, walking through nature not only a pleasure but a proven aid to general wellbeing, a stress-buster, a booster to both creativity and immune system function.

Walking, like a safe home, is also a primal urge; we didn't evolve to be upright on two legs for nothing. It's what makes us the world's top predator, alongside the inventions of fire, tools and mass cooperation. It's known to increase blood flow, flood your brain with dopamine and serotonin, create 'divergent thinking' and sophisticated cognitive abilities, stimulate interaction between the two brain hemispheres (the logical left and the intuitive right) and thus make your brain actually *grow*. Microsoft's Bill Gates is, and Apple's Steve Jobs was, a dedicated walker, the latter famously holding walking meetings to encourage free-flowing ideas, the kind of ideas which, you know, change the world for ever. Walking, science tells us, raises our pain threshold and improves mood, self-esteem and calm. It decreases depression, anger, anxiety, frustration and hostility (all of which, sadly, define much of the twenty-first century so far).

In literature, The Greats have known the benefits of walking for centuries. Dickens walked up to ten miles around London for inspiration most days while Nietzsche once intoned, grandly, 'All truly great thoughts are conceived by walking.' Several iconic authors, from Ernest Hemingway to J. K. Rowling, have declared walking the only reliable cure for writer's block.

Millions of us, throughout the bizarre, shocking, often deadly two years of the pandemic, took to our legs and strode away from home, the daily pound often the only respite from enclosed walls and enforced claustrophobia. For me, certainly, through the most miserable weeks of spring 2020, the daily walk became my daily sense-of-achievement, when often nothing else could be achieved, other than a lunchtime intake of a fridge-cooled mound of unsalted egg mayonnaise. I could time the upswing in mood: twenty minutes into the upwards stride, as the views across London began stretching out below, came a palpable surge of positive energy, of belief in future wellness, of delight in the season's new thrills.

During these two years Chris Packham, the sometime troubled boy with Asperger's, never tired of telling us how much nature is both an emotional and psychological healer, his own life literally saved by wetlands, wildlife and poodles.

In early summer 2020, trapped in the hospital treatment chair, it was to Chris Packham I turned, now taking his duty as public broadcaster so seriously and enthusiastically he created a half-hour online, guerrilla naturalist show with his stepdaughter Megan McCubbin called *The Self-Isolating Bird Club*, beamed from the New Forest and watched every day by 7.8 million people. This led to their appearance together on 2020's best-ever series of *Springwatch*, followed by their *Springwatch* midday offshoot *Out To Lunch*. Sitting in that reclining chemo chair, legs up, poison pouring into my bloodstream via the excellent port, time drifted soothingly by while marvelling at the lifestyle of the ink-black stag beetle and its majestically deadly antlers. That summer, Chris Packham had much to say about the situation our planet suddenly faced.

'Speaking entirely biologically,' he announced in June 2020, 'what the whole, horribly harsh, tragic lesson of the virus has taught us is that we are part of nature; we're not there to hold dominion over it, we're not above it. A global conversation about how many people the planet can sustain is something that has to happen. We've always been exposed to pathogens – everything from smallpox to bubonic plague. We've beaten them through our advances in science and I'm not regretting that. But we are an organism, living on a planet, and the way we were living was unsustainable. We were overcrowded, we were eating animals that we'd shipped alive from one part of the world to another and we're paying a terrible price for it. Let's be honest: a lot of the governments that have mishandled the corona crisis are not going to survive it. I sincerely hope that there will be a huge peaceful shake-up and people will start moving in the right direction.'

More evidence, then, that the people who become politicians (in this era, certainly) are exactly the kind of people who should never become politicians or be given the power to run much more than the spin cycle on a washing machine.

When we first moved into our flat on the park's edge, I was the kind of person who'd always get the bus, or an actual *cab*, back from the pub in Crouch End or Muswell Hill, both maximum 20-minute walks. Today, the only time I ever do so is when the weather is atrocious or it's the depths of danger-zone night. For years, and especially the last two, I've walked everywhere, whether the four miles there and back to hospital or the two miles to the nearby woods of Highgate on a weekend, where we stroll around and listen out, ears like satellite dishes, for the rare sound, and maybe even sight, of an overhead drilling woodpecker. It's been a lifestyle change shared by millions during the global tragedy which shrunk our lives: the smaller they became, the more we engaged with the big outdoors, every day, not least those who suddenly found themselves strolling round parklands with a dog, or even two.

Those Healing Nature Vibes we've heard so much about are, if anything, underestimated. It's not just the peace or the beauty, not just the rapture of ecosystems or the joy of regeneration, or even the fact our lives are so short and fragile in the face of a single two-hundred-year-old oak tree; it's the immersion in a different realm from the rest of the contemporary world. Nature wants nothing from us (other than to leave it alone), it's not trying to sell us anything, turn us into addicts in the name of commerce, lie to us for its own ends, fuel our insecurities, judge us, scam us, spam us, or violently attack and kill us. Other than when it does in, say, a climate-change-induced natural disaster, in which case we only have ourselves to blame.

Back in 1991, when myself and Jill visited Ali in Sydney, we waved her goodbye in the big city where she was working for a year and went walkabout through east coast Australia – or, rather, bus-about: we'd booked ourselves a three-week, hop-on/hop-off bus route through many small towns and hostels-in-the-wilderness, where you were expected to stay a few days before the next bus picked you up. But we always took the same bus onwards the following morning because, er, I fancied the bus driver, much to Jill's bewilderment (and to zero romantic avail). Arriving at our final destination, Cairns, Queensland, we headed for the boats which take you to the Barrier Reef, where we booked a five-day diving trip. Jill was already a certified scuba diver; I would merely be allowed to snorkel. I'd never snorkelled, I'd no idea what to expect. I wasn't expecting a *completely different planet*.

Just below the surface of the ocean lies the teeming kaleidoscopic coral, bursting with creatures you've only seen via David Attenborough, creatures of a thousand different shapes more beautiful and curious than anything we've ever conjured through the imagination of science-fiction. So many huge eyes, searching tendrils and neon stripes; a wavy-winged ray, a shimmering shoal of electric blue tiddlers surrounding you, a purple-and-gold butterflyfish bobbing past your face with its elongated snout, blithely ignoring the foot-splashing monster among them, scooshing together through the gently wafting anemones in rainbow colours, in a world which has existed for twenty million years. Tears trickled from my eyes, pooling at the bottom of my mask. The aliens are already among us. And they come in peace.

One night, as Jill and the divers splashed backwards overboard on a night dive, the skipper, a Captain Birdseye character, invited me up the ladder to the topmost platform for an aerial view, pointing into the sky. There it was: the Milky Way, directly above our heads, the vast, curving sweep blazing in blues, yellows, orange and mauve, this spiral galaxy we're all living inside, the cap'n expertly pointing out the Southern Cross, the pointer stars of Alpha and Beta Centauri, talking about star clouds and nebulae and the red giant star Betelgeuse as I'm standing there, in the balmy still of an Australian December summer, aged twenty-six, wondering how we ever managed to get here, two kids from small-town Scotland with heads full of travelling dreams.

This wasn't another planet, this was *our* planet. We've never needed the obscene coffers of the billionaires to take us to the edge of space, we're already in outer space. We always have been.

It's a thought which has never left me, the biggest Big Picture thought of them all. A thought that's needed more than ever when your world has never felt so small.

20

THINGS CAN ONLY GET BETTER

A week after the constipation calamity on Hitler's birthday, as the April sunshine glimmers on in the park, there's an incident with the opposite problem: yet another Bathroom Humiliation, once again witnessed by Simon. I feel inconsolably sad, not just for my own situation but for him, a man who has now witnessed things no life partner, no soul mate, no *lover* ever should.

I've a hospital appointment with Dr Bridger later today and don't know how I'll make the two-mile walk without a desperate need for the toilet. I'm too virus-nervous, still, to travel by bus. On *Good Morning Britain*, a report begins about an elderly war veteran in a care home and his 17-year-old carer, who gives him a gift of his late wife's face on a cushion, which he embraces as if she's alive, kissing the silken image. It's a happy, romantic, sad, all-too-human story and it makes me uncontrollably weep. I'm standing in the kitchen crying when Simon walks in.

'What's wrong?'

'This is all just ... *horrible*.'

We fold ourselves into each other's arms.

This will end, this will end, this will end.

I make it to Doc Bridger without public incident. There's been little improvement with the mouth ulcers so she's again reducing the dose of this latest chemo. It's partly what they mean by 'tailor-made' treatments, tinkering not only with what you need, but what you can reasonably tolerate.

'We'll keep going,' she tells me, 'do whatever we can to get you to the end.' The whole point of this weekly chemo is to eradicate as many lurking sinister cells as possible, to stop the cancer coming back. They're already trying to save me in the future, to help me live as long as I possibly can. Unlike the measures President Trump is now advocating to supposedly save the citizens of America: the injecting of disinfectant as the answer to Covid. God *help* America!

With the new reduced dose things begin to stabilise, slowly. With tiny mouth improvements I can feel and see the healing process, the miracle of our self-healing bodies, as regenerative as the leaves on the tree outside our window. Within weeks I feel so normal it feels *abnormal*. I'm ecstatic, reminded once again how normality is all we ever need, normality *is* The Miracle. I can *actually eat*. A bowl of pasta with mushroom 'n' cream sauce is so delicious it makes me cry. For the first time in what feels like years – it's certainly been months – I find I'm singing out loud, cleaning the fridge when a Gerry Cinnamon song begins frolicking inside my head, with lyrics musing on never thinking you'd make it this far. It's the week Captain Tom near Bedford has officially raised almost forty million pounds for the NHS and is currently No. 1 in the UK charts, with Michael Ball and 'You'll Never Walk Alone'. The best of us, as ever, appearing at the worst of times.

By early May we're braving a trip to Muswell Hill, where everything remains closed except the coffee shops. We buy takeaway coffees for the first time all year and sit down, with some excitement, on a public bench. My creamy flat white is *beyond delicious*. And hot! The weekly treatments carry on, mouth tenderness comes and goes, but nothing stops me functioning. I'm now only partially ill and partially ill I can do. Walking through the park, everything is so green, so beautiful, so bursting with woodland life it feels like a psychedelic drug experience without The Fear. There's even talk of Covid restrictions lifting for the summer. It's all going to be all right.

Isn't it?

All through May 2020 there's not a drop of rain, perfect late spring conditions. At the many offices of No. 10 Downing Street on Wednesday 20th, one hundred people are invited to bring their own booze to a garden shindig to 'make the most of the lovely weather', while the rest of us plebs are forbidden from meeting more than one other person outside. We don't know that at the time, of course, it's incendiary information several No. 10 insiders will sit on for most of the next two years, including Boris Johnson's chief advisor Dominic Cummings.

Five days after thirty to forty No.10 insiders were 'making the most of the lovely weather', Dominic Cummings is forced to explain his Covid-rule-flouting drive to Barnard Castle 'to test his eyesight' in a press conference in the No. 10 rose garden. A withering reception and many jokes about Specsavers ensue. Cummings plays the long game, the soon-to-be-ousted advisor then biding his time for maximum 'partygate' exposé carnage in early 2022. Over in America, meanwhile, a black man called George Floyd is murdered in front of the planet by a white copper's knee. The world, it certainly feels, is about to blow up.

The postponed MRI scan finally goes ahead, followed by a Doc Bridger consultation. The tumour has shrunk but there's 'footprint activity in the breast which the chemo won't cure'. And so, the confirmation comes: a lumpectomy won't be enough and the breast must be removed. It's what I was expecting anyway. Dates are set: end of chemo 25 June, if all goes to plan; 9 July for surgery.

The surgeon rings with 'good news': in these surgically

compromised Covid times she's pleased she can offer me a breast reconstruction on the day of the mastectomy. I'm called in to see her and assistant Martha, who come as a surgical duo, the pair close colleagues who constantly amuse each other and always admire whatever idiotic, fluorescent footwear I happen to be wearing that day. I'm to be given a breast implant called an expander, a surgical process where the outer skin of the breast (without my long-binned nipple) will be kept – 'spared', as it's known – under which a sling-type device will hold an implant in place. The implant itself has a silicone outer skin hosting silicone gel or saline, attached to a port fitted under the skin, from which more gel can be injected, or syphoned out, depending on weight gain and loss. They log my height and weight. I'm now 55.2 kg, eight and a half stone and, somehow, an inch shorter, at five foot five and a half. Swizzed yet again!

By late June, chemo is over *at last*. While I wait for surgery, a celebration is planned. I'm going to drink booze again. And eat crisps again. I feel elated: it's the most I've had to look forward to in six months. Ev has dropped off a Glasto Swag Bag for the Glastonbury weekend that doesn't exist this year, including two cans of Strongbow. I can't wait, literally, and on the sunny Thursday afternoon, with Simon, take her two cans and one family-sized bag of chicken-flavoured crisps to the uplands of Ally Pally.

I hear the tantalising *pssssssst!* of the Strongbow ring-pull for the first time since Christmas 2019, take a sip and … *euerrrgh!* My beloved cider tastes like petrol. It's undrinkable, a wash of toxic, fumy chemicals I cannot tolerate. I try a few crisps … *aiiieeeee!* A handful of chicken crisps feels like a mouthful of needles, my mouth too raw and ravaged, still, to deal with this jagged intrusion. I abandon Project Glasto.

Beyond swizzed again.

I was nowhere near ready, it turns out, mouth now disintegrating again, an ulcer on the tongue, one in the back of the throat. All foods hurt again to varying degrees, even a drink of *still* water stings. But my last chemo is done. I made it to cycle No. 11 and the poisons will now begin, gradually, to ebb away.

Countdown to The Chop begins.

21

DRY YER EYES MATE

Ali's had a phrase for decades which translates as, 'Let's go to the pub.' She simply says, 'Put yer eyebrows on.' When my eyebrows are on, I'm going OUT.

As eyebrows go, they aren't especially shapely – fairly thinnish, average – but when I sharpen an eyebrow pencil and draw on a better pair – thicker, darker, with angled edges – they act as a kind of Superwoman Shield, or even antlers. Totems, however illusory, of confidence, maturity and being up for the fight and flight of everyday life. As a sometime natural blonde I've always had unusually dark brown eyebrows, easily exploited into cartoon-level contours. Siouxsie Sioux, of course, made me do it, back in '79 as a fledgling post-punk believer, even if her level of mythologically powerful, sphinx-like drama could never be reached by the likes of me.

Now, in 2020, I have no eyebrows. There's a *suggestion* of eyebrows there, wispy, ghostly echoes of a lifetime's facial characteristic, now all but obliterated by chemotherapy. But when I'm going out (which in Covid times means, glamorously, the hospital, park or supermarket), I *still* draw them on, even though the effect is less Siouxsie Sioux, more Bette Davis in *Whatever Happened to Baby Jane?* With no guiding line and no sturdy hair for the crayon to build on, only the bare bump above the eye socket, it's just a line drawn on skin over bone. Mine is not a big head either, it's curiously small and now the edges are all sticking out, the cheekbones, jaw and brow ridge. For the first time ever, I can clearly see that my head is *a human skull*. You don't want to acknowledge that your head is a human skull because skulls, usually, are something dusty in the hand of an archaeologist or attached to a skeleton in a TV sitcom surgery or to someone who is definitely dead, already in their coffin and heading into the crematorium flames. This, surely, is how I'd look if I was on my deathbed today, at the age of fifty-five: identical to my mother on her deathbed, aged seventy-four.

I've no eyelashes either. Sometimes, walking in the park, a flying insect will hurtle into a lash-free open eye and drown, resulting in face-contorting eye-twitches and bending over double, trying to swill away the remnants with a dripping palmful of hastily poured drinking water. We know what eyelashes are primarily for – a barrier against incoming irritants, the eyes' first line of defence – and yet we spend billions coating them in potential irritants, in the form of mascara (ingredients include iron oxide pigment, castor oil and paraffin) to 'achieve' the Bambi-eyed look, because we're programmed to find it attractive, in ourselves and everyone else. To this end I've personally contributed to the beauty industry billions via the regular purchase of jet-black L'Oréal 'volumiser' mascaras for over forty years (even before I knew I was supposedly 'worth it'). But when you have no eyelashes, unlike eyebrows, you can't draw them on. And false eyelashes on a skull only works for Halloween.

In the bathroom mirror, post-shower, with what's left of my hair swept back and damp, Edvard Munch's *The Scream* stares back at me. The once regularly highlighted, shiny blonde hair is the most sparse, dull and shapeless it has ever been. Even with the rigours of the cold cap I've lost a third of my hair and it's naturally thin anyway; today, a drab, unkempt, threadbare, mousy-brown ruin, bald at the sides where the cap couldn't clamp, like the fright-wig of an itinerant eighties' crustie, with visible thinning on top. I've followed the instructions for months: wash sparingly, no colouring whatsoever until treatment is fully over. My nails are chemo-ruined, too, currently made of paper and painfully torn, deep into the quick (all Sellotape edge-finding endeavours, for several months, are impossible).

The good news is I don't have to bother shaving my legs any more. There's nothing there to shave. The pubic hair, too, in case you're wondering (I really hope you're not wondering), is barely there, at best a sorry comb-over like Archie Gemmill's in the Scotland football team in 1978. Not that there's much going on down there anyway: chemotherapy robs your libido, all right. No wonder: puckering up with a mouthful of fungal ulcerations, for a start, isn't anyone's idea of erotica (unless you're seriously unhinged).

Watching TV at home one day an ad comes on for mascara. I blink with my lash-less eyes and wonder why it was that I used to care so much about the concept of luscious lashes. Did I care that much? I don't think I really did, it's just something we do, because we can, because attraction is central to the life-force. You just want to feel, you know, as reasonably attractive as you can with the raw materials given. Which has always made me feel sorry for (most) blokes, because the face they wake up with is as good as it's going to get for the rest of the day.

I know now, though, that I do not care about my eyelashes or my eyebrows any more. I'm not crushed, depressed or bereft, grieving for any aspect of bodily hair. Yes, I look like an alien, but I won't look like this for ever, and without the science that's making me look like an alien I would soon be dead instead. Simon, who is not blind, doesn't even mention the physical changes, other than the Boney P quip, but no eyebrows or eyelashes, mousy-brown hair and a sticky-out jawline is the least he's had to feel sad about only a few months on from imagining scattering my ashes round the base of 'our' tree in Ally Pally Park.

Much more than chin-quivering nostalgia for what's been lost, in fact, the mascara ad seems brazenly absurd, starring young women who are beautiful and almost certainly digitally enhanced, with lashes as lengthy as clothes poles. We're all beautiful when we're young anyway because youth *is* beautiful. We all know, when we see photos of our youthful selves, how it truly is wasted on the young.

All makeup, hair, skincare and beauty product ads, from this day on, appear as flagrant mockery to me, the multi-billion-pound global beauty industry so obviously toying with every one of us, so blatantly contributing to the sum of human misery, to the contemporary insecurity catastrophe, the one we're more willing, every year, to both facilitate and spectacularly fund. Under the pretext of progressive 'science' – all state-of-the-art microbiomes, cryotherapy, prebiotics and 'cleanical skincare' – humanity has 'evolved' to psychologically obliterate itself with unfounded fears over the thinnest, outermost layer of ourselves when all we need is for our bodies to work. They know it. *We* know it. And yet, wilfully, we live in the age of *Love Island*, of Madonna's new head, of cosmetic surgery clinics inundated with requests for extreme distortion 'maximalism' procedures, heart-shaped 'Russian lips' and the 2021-coined 'alienised' look – as artificially concocted for Angelina Jolie's *Maleficent* character, with shelf-like cheekbones and abnormally arched eyebrows (save yourself a fortune, chums, and opt for a life-threatening disease instead).

A Marc Jacobs perfume ad champions the opposite of alien and disturbs me just as much, the one for 'Perfect', featuring today's requisite diverse spectrum of what appears to be normal young women, which most of them are, chosen from a social media casting call alongside a few models, including Kate Moss's daughter Lila.

'I'm perfect,' beams one, before everyone else joins in: 'I'm perfect' … 'I'm perfect' … 'I'm perfect'.

Not so very long ago, we grew up with a much kinder truism, and one which is actually true. 'Nobody's perfect.' Because nobody is, and nobody ever was. As a word 'perfect' should be binned, surely, from the context of human physicality. I've never once believed I am or could be or even wanted to be 'perfect'. I don't even know what perfect *means*. I do know it doesn't exist, other than, er, in perfect numbers and something called perfect maths. It might be definable to some, of course, through the filtered illusions on their Instagram feeds, but we all know where that leads: demolished mental health. I've spent decades in conversation with The Beautiful People, throughout music, film and TV, heard many testimonials on the nature of beauty from celebrated beauties themselves, female and male, from Beyoncé, Mel Gibson and Nicole Kidman, to Keira Knightly, Hugh Jackman and Mila Kunis. Every one of these disparate characters dismissed their own physical beauty as mere 'luck' and certainly no priority: they cared about the work, relationships, success, family, fulfilment. Of course, they *would* say that, to spare we mortals more neuroses, but the women especially would follow up such dismissals with a variation on this rueful snort, 'C'mon, what you're looking at on-screen/in the magazines? Even *I* can't live up to that!'

In the mirror, Edvard Munch's *The Scream* still stares back at me. I can't say I'm thrilled, but I can't say I'm heading for a PTSD diagnosis either. Or my own new head full of fillers (even if I could afford one). Maybe, I muse one day, it's to do with having seen dead bodies. There's nothing quite like the electrocuting sight of a dead body to make you profoundly realise what you thought you already knew, but you didn't really, not *for definite*: that this thing on the outside of ourselves, this swaddling cocoon of skin, all the stuff you can see, is only the human-shaped holdall that carries you, nothing to do with what makes you *you*, in all your complicated, miraculous uniqueness.

In 2004, staring down at my white-haired mother's alabaster body, translucent skin like parchment in her white floral nightie, she looked six hundred years old, a delicate, faded sketch from a Renaissance fresco, beautiful in its way and nothing to do with her. Nothing to do with *her* at all. This physical mass of skin and bone and muscle and water didn't encase her any more, didn't matter any more and ultimately never did. *She* just didn't exist any more. Even if, when I got back to her deafeningly silent empty home that afternoon, a large golden can of L'Oréal's Elnett hairspray, the kind she'd used for over forty years, still did.

But having no eyebrows, eyelashes, nails or a decent hairdo, is hardly a life-altering scenario. It's temporary for a start. Unlike having a breast sliced off for ever.

22

LESS THAN A WOMAN

Before you can be treated in any hospital in these Covid times, you must have first taken a nurse-administered Covid test forty-eight hours previously and, in the case of my treatments and forthcoming major surgery, a blood test too.

The Covid-swamped Northern has outsourced its cancer surgery, so this means a trip to a private hospital on the outskirts of London. In a day-patient side room, after tests and lengthy form-filling, I'm unexpectedly given a packet of Chlorhexidine Wash Cloths, its packaging heralding 'Large antiseptic body-cleansing cloths' (and furthermore), 'Rinse-free and moisturising rapid bacterial action, residual protection'. Illustrated instructions on the back tell me specifically where to wet wipe my body: 'Neck and torso, back, left arm and axilla, right arm and axilla, left leg and foot, right leg and foot, buttocks, groin' – i.e. everything except your head. The nurse tells me I must use these wipes the night before the mastectomy, though doesn't explain why: no one's going near my legs, feet, buttocks or groin, as far as I'm aware. Presumably, then, it's to expunge any plebian bacterial residue from my unhygienic skin before sliding into the four-thousand-thread count Egyptian cotton sateen bed sheets, the ones draped upon the bed whose previous occupant was second cousin to the 15th Marquess of Shrewsbury.

Before bedtime, I have a shower, dry off and apply the all-over wipes. Within minutes, I'm stinging all over, an itchy, rashy sting, not only in tender crevices but everywhere, as if the population of the wasps' nest living inside my mouth has suddenly escaped and is now dive-bombing in glee all around my body. I have another shower and scrub away the offending chemicals. Maybe it's a ruse, I'm now thinking, to make we freeloading NHS lowlifes have *two* showers.

Mastectomy Day, 9 July 2020.

After a 5.30 a.m. wake-up call, Simon drops me off in an Uber at 7 a.m. at the main entrance to the hospital where he can set no foot across the threshold. 'This is the line!' barks a masked door inspector, as he points a temperature gun at my head, instructs me to gel my hands while robotically asking, 'Have you had a recurring cough, runny nose, loss of taste and smell ...' He then reaches a gloved hand towards my nose, pinches in the still-straight wire at the top of my fresh surgical mask, no 'Excuse me' while he's at it.

I must register, talking through a Perspex screen with a clearly disinterested admin staffer seated in a booth. She asks for my name, address and then, already, '... and regarding payment?' My heart lurches. Seeing my fear, and possibly my thirteen-pound charity-shop raincoat, she asks, 'Are you through the NHS?' She takes my NHS hospital number, now even less interested, sliding under the screen a form I must fill where my mobile phone number has been printed incorrectly.

'Your surgeon,' she now asks. 'What's his first name?'

'She is ... a she.'

'Oh.'

Another staffer takes me to my private room, in silence, and I see hand sanitisers everywhere, along the corridors, in every room, bolted either side of the lifts, necessary, yes, but also a rigorous exercise in litigation avoidance. It's the first hour of my stay in this alien environment but the staff here have been markedly less friendly than they've been, without fail, at the Northern.

The door opens on my unknowably expensive private hospital room, not all that much more spacious than the standard NHS side rooms but here, from floor to ceiling, are door-sized windows, flooding the room with soothing, natural light. There's a desk and fabric-covered seat, as you'd find in a hotel suite, with a large oval mirror and a flat screen TV positioned on the wall above. The bed is not a hotel bed, it's a regulation hospital bed, secured on enormous castors. In the en suite bathroom, where the light works, there's a selection of miniature hand gels and hand creams (Templespa), exactly as you'd find in a hotel, in a room I suspect costs significantly more than Claridge's.

Within an hour my Northern surgeons arrive, Ms Jana and Martha (consultants often work across both private and NHS hospitals), bustling into the room full of chatter behind their masks, Martha marvelling at today's stupid shoes (black, platform, plastic boots with fluorescent yellow laces). With my top and bra off, Ms Jana draws lines with marker pen all over my right breast, an arrow also pointing upwards on my inner right arm to indicate which breast is for the scalpel (just in case). They bound out again and I stare at my two bare breasts in the bathroom mirror for the very last time. Perky is not the word. Fifty-five is more like the word. But they've served me well. I was never a 'tits-out' type anyway, even in my teens and twenties. More likely to be wearing a psychedelic shirt, grandad's cardigan and a geezer's classic raincoat. Having one breast does not matter to me, not today anyway. All that matters is staying alive. And the reconstruction will be OK, won't it?

A series of nurses appear with various forms and questions. I don't need to sign a 'possibility of pregnancy' form because I'm through the menopause. Half an hour later another nurse arrives with the same form, which I now must sign because, despite what

I've said, I'm still in the pregnancy age range (somehow). Another nurse takes my blood pressure, an incoming doctor wonders what the readings were, asks if one is under a hundred, to which the nurse says 'No,' and I have to correct her: 'It's eighty-six!' I'm given a pair of control socks which are both left feet. I'm given a menu (a proper menu) and the dates are wrong, it's the ninth, where it says the eleventh, alongside a discharge date of the eleventh.

Soon, wearing the same regulation, diamond-motif gown as the NHS, I'm escorted to the surgical ward, and placed on a surgery table where several strangers in masks crowd around my soon-to-be sliced apart body. A cannula is secured in the back of my left hand. It's frightening; no one introduces themselves, until the anaesthetist makes herself known. A nurse places a blood pressure cuff around my left upper arm and then holds my left wrist alarmingly tightly, pressing my cannula'd hand down on the table. The anaesthetist approaches with a needle, injects a potion and I'm suddenly screaming out loud, my upper body bolting upright, a burning pain of intense magnitude shooting upwards, as if my arm has been electrocuted by lightning. The last thing I remember before passing out is a nurse shouting, 'Oh no!' as she releases the blood pressure cuff, which was mistakenly left at full inflation as the anaesthetic was injected. So much for gently 'drifting off'. Ali will tell me later this is a dangerous cock-up (the circulation cut off, constricting the blood vessels) which no one in this private hospital will ever acknowledge or apologise for and I don't have the heart to complain about. I'm too grateful for all my treatment. But I'm pretty sure the toffs, paying thousands, would.

Post-surgery I wake up in my room. There's a tube inserted into my upper right body, an inch under the reconstructed breast – which is covered with a huge dressing – leading to a large plastic bottle on the floor, into which blood from the wound will regularly drip.

In the oval mirror opposite the bed my curiously blue-grey

face is poking out from the bedsheets. I must go to the loo and can't move, can't manoeuvre upwards, the pain throughout my right torso is unbearable. I reach, slowly, for the nurse alert button dangling beside the bed and one immediately appears, gingerly pulls me upwards, and forward, off the bed and onto my feet, now shuffling me forward while I grip onto her arm, all the way to the loo. She's the first kind and gentle nurse I've met in here.

Two other nurses soon march in, one declaring, 'What's happened in here ... a war!?', motioning to a pile of medical paraphernalia that's been dumped on the floor in front of the bed: calf clamps, tubes, cloths. As boombastic reggae dude Shaggy once said: it wasn't me. The other nurse takes the obs, jabbing the thermometer gun unnecessarily sharply deep inside my ear. Another nurse yanks hard on my drain tube, the one attached to my body, declaring, 'What's this!?', as if she's no idea why I'm in here. A nurse taking a blood test asks me if it's OK to use the right arm, on the side of the surgery, as if I'm supposed to know. I'm told things are about to happen, which then don't happen for an hour, like the bringing of water or the attachment of a fluid drip. When the water comes, it's in a heavy steel jug, which I can't lift up with either arm, it's too painful. A nurse fills a glass for me, in haste, and the glass spills over, splashing all over the bedclothes. Someone else arrives with what appears to be an actual hotel dinner menu, featuring a spectrum of delicious options, and stands silently over me like an intimidating border control officer with a headset and clipboard at Los Angeles airport.

If there had been one cold staff member, one rough nurse or one incident of ineptitude, I would understand – these people are very busy. But this has been relentless, a catalogue of careless, uncaring individuals and sometimes serious incompetence, something I'd experienced nowhere in the NHS, where I'd been met by effortless warmth and compassion, day after day, for seven months. We're hardwired in the UK to evangelise about the NHS, and more so than ever in the year 2020, but this is an unexpected revelation. The NHS staff are simply much better at their jobs than the ones in this private hospital on every level imaginable: faster, kinder, far more focused, knowledgeable, calming.

I have a theory. The hospital staff in the private sector are so used to complaints, to being barked at and ordered around by the wealthy and entitled, they've learned to keep patients at arm's length. And resent them for it. I've heard things which back it up: I'm wearing electronic cuffs wrapped around my calves, which make them feel like they're being massaged, pressure running slowly up and down, inflating and relaxing, making constant bleeping noises. This is a blood clot prevention device, state of the art, and important. One of the friendlier nurses tells me some patients call this 'torture', and refuse to wear them, which causes the nurses much admin time with waiver forms, lest litigation happen if someone dies from a clot. The nurse tells me her friend died from a blood clot aged twenty-one.

It seems obvious, really. They're used to berks in here, rude people, the staff mostly young people living in London on salaries doubtless swallowed up by extortionate rented flats at the unsavoury end of a tube line. One nurse asks where I live. She hasn't heard of Hornsey: not many have. But she's heard of Alexandra Palace. 'That's a nice area,' she says, and behind her mask I hear nothing but sadness.

I switch on the flat screen TV and watch *Celebrity Masterchef*, where Phil Daniels is a contestant, the man who will for ever be, to me and my pals, Jimmy out of 1979's *Quadrophenia*. This is the character who set the template, for me at least, of never having A Proper Job and rejecting the workplace hierarchy (inviting a lifetime of financial turmoil). A pivotal scene from the film remains indelible in my mind, the one where Jimmy's boss in the post office finds his absenteeism intolerable, tells him many lads his age would give their eye teeth for a steady job like this.

'Find one, then!' retorts Jimmy. 'I'll tell you what you can do with your eye teeth and your job – you can take that mail and that franking machine and all that other rubbish I have to go about with and you can stuff 'em right up your arse!'

Forty-one years after that scene first penetrated my fourteen-year-old mind, rearranged my synapses and laid down the paving stones of the yellow brick road of the future, 'Jimmy' was on *Masterchef* and I was lying in a hospital bed with a life-threatening disease, tubes hanging out from surgical holes, with a blue face and an alien protrusion stuck to the front of my body. I text my *Quadrophenia*-loving friends and how we all laugh, rumly.

The food in this hospital is not beamed from the 1970s. It's beamed from what tastes like a five-star hotel kitchen in 2020 and I've chosen a delicious three-course meal: lentil soup, baked salmon, broccoli, boiled potatoes, sweet potato fries and a raspberry tart with the plate artfully swiped in flavour-popping raspberry coulis. The procedure I'm having today, by itself (never mind all the other treatments), would privately cost between six and seven thousand pounds, and in my experience for significantly less competent care: the food, then, is really all you're paying for – one hell of an expensive meal. (Here endeth the lesson, comrades.)

I'm here for one night only, perhaps all the NHS can afford, discharged the following morning with the drainage bottle filling with sporadically dripping blood. I'm given a large paper pharmacy bag full of painkillers and leaflets detailing gentle exercises to offset worrisome conditions called 'roping' and 'seroma'. A hospital business partner (apparently a registered charity) selling post-mastectomy swimwear has also provided a home time goody bag: a packet of Eton Mess gourmet sweets, a bag of beef Hula Hoops, a hand and lip-balm combo, a glossy swimwear brochure and a fetching grey, polka-dot Drain Dollies tote bag – designed to bring a fashionable touch to the lugging of an urn of blood. The drainage bottle now nestles inside the Drain Dolly, nattily worn over the shoulder, while the tube of blood dangles below my coat. Ev and Simon are waiting in the car park, staring, as I appear through the front door like an extra in *Shaun of the Dead*, inching so slowly the new national hero Captain Tom and his walking frame would whizz straight past me as if driving an F1 McLaren.

Simon puts my overnight bag in the boot while Ev helps me into the car. It's a fair step up to the front passenger seat, so she holds onto the contents of the Drain Dolly, inside which she can clearly see a large plastic bottle swilling with deep red blood. She is very squeamish about blood, has even fainted at the sight of a needle. We set off and she laughs ruefully: 'I can't believe I've just had to hold a bottle of your blood. We're a long way from The Sally now.'

23

DANCE YOURSELF DIZZY

We're on the dancefloor of The Sally, Perth's Salutation Hotel, as in *on the floor*, sitting down, legs splayed out in Vs, bunched up against whichever chum or stranger is sitting down in front of us, joining in on the world's most ludicrous dance craze. We're in rows upon lengthy rows, thirty people long, stretching along the dancefloor, arms out wide leaning over to the right, leaning over to the left, tapping on the floor to the funkin' beats of The Gap Band's 'Oops Upside Your Head'. Now, we're doing the shoulder shimmy, forward and back, forward and back, rowing without paddles, side to side again, clapping overhead, a little bit more to the right, a little bit more to the left, in increasingly acute angles until the whole seated conga line of disco-berserk buffoons have keeled over in a limb-entangled heap.

The Four of Us are fifteen years old and The Sally, a nightclub supposedly for over-eighteens, is letting us in (for now). Our fringes are damp, our mascara run, from the hours and hours of proper dancing, not in a heap on the floor but spinning and jiving and twisting to the disco tunes of a delirious 1980, to Ottowan's 'D.I.S.C.O', Kelly Marie's 'Feels Like I'm in Love', the Detroit Spinners' 'Working My Way Back to You'. The silver glitterball dazzles overhead, strobe lights in primary colours shoot like sabres across the room. 'Only when I'm dancing can I feel this free,' squeaked Madonna back in '85 and in nine swift, simple words defined the very nature of this primal, powerful, instinctive human need for physical, emotional and existential abandon.

We've all danced for ever, me and my friends, as most of us do, through all the decades and all the countries, towns and cities we've ever lived in or holidayed in; this constant, communal pleasure we humans are born to do. From the under-eighteens discos at Perth's Lesser City Hall, to the St Albans mod revival club where myself, Ali, Rimmy and Jill bounced around the floor in a stand-up conga line to the 'nutty, nutty sound' of Madness, to the disco fevers of the Wheel Inn. By 1980 my black-and-white mod uniform had exploded into technicolour pandemonium: a flamingo-pink seersucker suit and matching pink shirt, gleefully non-matched with fluorescent yellow satin gloves, sweating and twirling as the disco hits kept coming: Liquid Gold's 'Dance Yourself Dizzy', Blondie's 'Atomic', Odyssey's 'Use It Up and Wear It Out', Lipps, Inc.'s irresistibly berserk 'Funky Town'.

The dancing never stopped, through the culturally tribal eras that followed in the bountiful early eighties, all those sounds and startling sights from the gaudy new romantics, spectral goths, art-school dandies and extravagantly bequiffed indie kids, present in abundance at Perth's Banana Club and in Scotland's best nightclub/venues, from the fabled Barrowlands in Glasgow to the Nite Club in Edinburgh to Fat Sam's in Dundee. Within those steamy walls a generation flailed in communal frenzy to the peacock parade of characters on stage, from Southern Death Cult, Siouxsie and the Banshees and Theatre of Hate, to Gene Loves Jezebel, Billy Mackenzie and The Smiths. The hairdos, too, of the provincial dancefloor devotees were as flamboyant and silly as the shape-throwing stars on *Top of the Pops*, from Adam Ant to Boy George to Morrissey.

In '83/'84, when myself, Jill and Ev lived together as school leavers in a two-bedroom, shoddily carpeted flat in central Perth, we were always going round the corner, to another hotel with a nightclub, The Grampian. On a Sunday it opened mid-afternoon, The Four of Us then lost for up to eight hours in a constant frug to Elvis Costello, Aztec Camera and The Bluebells, after which loitering reprobates came back to ours for parties fuelled by cider and Pernod, where we'd dreamily waft to the unfathomable phonetics of the Cocteau Twins' 'Pearly Dewdrops Drop'. Once, some hapless hobo fell asleep on our living-room couch and pissed himself. The stink lingered for weeks.

The dancing carried on, through the early London years and acid house era of the late eighties, in fields until dawn, through the early nineties, in myriad London clubs: Syndrome, where Alex and Dave from Blur ever-frolicked under the spotlights; the Heavenly Sunday Social in the Albany pub basement, where table-top dancing erupted via DJs the Dust Brothers (soon Chemical Brothers); Blow Up in Camden, where the next generation of mods danced on the snooker table; and Smashing, where Jarvis Cocker spun on the lit-up seventies' panelled dancefloor as featured in Pulp's 'Disco 2000'. Britpop singalongs and superstar DJs then dominated every festival, while the 2000s brought the Big Pop mainstream club-night thrillers, from Beyoncé to Girls Aloud. At a *Glamour* magazine awards ceremony in 2008 – the mag's high-gloss, annual shindig featuring free booze all night – I took to the dancefloor, as I always did, at the first throb of the bassline in Michael Jackson's 'Billie Jean'. This time, I was unfathomably attempting to mimic the style of the dance duo on that year's *Britain's Got Talent*, Signature, whose 'Billie Jean' moves involved hopping on one leg while jiggling the other jubilantly in the air. Naturally, I fell over, crashed onto the floor and fractured three ribs, which took months to heal. No guts, no glory, I guess.

Today, though, leaving club life to the young, it's all about the kitchen disco, both at home and in the homes of friends, leaping round islands and Formica-topped tables to the sound of whatever those present have hollered in the vague direction of Alexa.

No wonder, when the dancing in public stopped in 2020, one of the emergent cultural triumphs was Sophie Ellis-Bextor's Kitchen Disco, turning her personal space into a Friday night club on Instagram, her exuberant kids tumbling around her feet. Throughout the UK and beyond, the planet was now kitchen-incarcerated, the only place where dancing could ever take place, whether in couples, family groups or in solo life with a cat. For two unforeseeably long years, despite the communal joy being shelved, the dancing proved not only unstoppable, but vital.

Through my own 2020, though, I wasn't doing much dancing, what with the blowtorched mouth, starvation and the permanent inner cold. I *really missed* the dancing. But after surgery in the summer of 2020, never mind perilous Billie Jean knees-up manoeuvres; for a while I was unable to even walk.

24

STUCK ON YOU

Christ! This hurts. The pain around the implant where my breast no longer exists is formidable, a gnawing, bone-deep ache meaning I can barely move. Painkillers are now a constant but I'm wary, with indelible memories of the constipation crisis. Ms Jana rings, urges me to take more painkillers, which I do even though the effects remain loathsome, back to that dozy half-life underwater. Seated on the sofa, legs up on a pouffe, nothing can be done except watch continuous episodes of the soothing, heroically humane *Repair Shop* on iPlayer.

The Drain Dolly is my constant companion, the tube still inserted into my body as I attempt to sleep. When the loo calls at 3 a.m. Simon must do what the kindly nurse did and let me grip onto his arm as he hauls me forward so I can slide out of bed, an undignified effort which gives me the one-eyed look, he tells me, of 'Thom Yorke from Radiohead'. It's the first time I've felt fully depressed through the whole experience. It's not just the exhaustion and the pain – there's been plenty of that already – it's that Simon, for the first time, really *does* feel like my carer now. He never complains, which only makes me even sorrier, even more crushed that our life together has become *this*. Without him, I can't even get out of bed. I'm useless, that dreaded word a '*burden*', for me a sobering insight into the hidden world of those who permanently care, and how their dependents must feel. No wonder we need professionals. How appalling they're paid a pittance.

Ali texts, which unleashes tears, so I ring her up, needing her to just talk to me, about how I'll be all right, about nonsense, which she does, and saves me. She then sends flowers, as does Leesa, two bountiful bunches I split and place around the flat, hoping to jolly the place up. Instead, it looks like I'm dead already and the funeral is imminent. The mouth ulcers are improving slightly but are still there, even one month after the end of chemo, a stinger on the roof of the mouth, another behind the upper lip.

Adding financial injury to all the other injuries, the only music magazine I now work for, *Q* – which has stoically and often brilliantly carried on through the pandemic even as the music industry buckled – is forced to fold in July 2020. The shockwaves of Covid have shunted it over the edge: no one is on tour, albums are pushed back, the life-support machine of advertising finally unplugged from an already dying publication. Its demise is announced, briefly, on ITV news on 20 July 2020, the last of the UK's physical, monthly, contemporary mainstream music magazines to die, after thirty-four years. RIP old pal, 1986–2020.

An appointment with Doc Bridger brings fresh developments. Biopsy tests on the breast they chopped off have found 'residual' cancer cell growth not killed off by all those months of chemo. They can't be certain there isn't more elsewhere in my body so there's further treatment to come.

I stare at her, aghast.

This finding is 'annoying', she adds, 'but we won't take any chances.' The good news is a new treatment has just become available on the NHS, given the financial go-ahead this May: it's a state-of-the-art, targeted chemotherapy that will attack specifically the kind of cancer cells I have. It works almost like an antibody, meaning it won't attack most of the rest of me, as the general chemo did. Which is just as well.

'It's for a year,' she tells me, 'but of course it's up to you.'

'A year? Chemo for another year!?'

'We wouldn't give it to anyone for that length of time if it wasn't something you could tolerate,' she assures. 'You won't even need the cold cap. There are still immune suppressant risks, you'll still have to be careful, but it's an incredible development and one that didn't exist only a few months ago.'

Once again, I'm seriously fortunate: the treatment, called Kadcyla, was not only not available until two months ago, but costs – for one course of treatment – £51,000. So once again, if I lived in America, *I would be doomed*.

The Kadcyla treatment begins, given every three weeks, back in the chemo suite, attached to the drip on the pole with the castors. Naturally, there's a different price to be paid, an irksome side effect known as neuropathy, where your feet and hands feel numb or tingly or occasionally even electrocuted, in my case always in the feet, as if thawing out from frostbite. It's caused by nerve damage and could be permanent. It's yet another condition that keeps me awake all night with shooting pains and spasms in my feet, the occasional electric shock jolting through a foot at 4 a.m. Taking Neurofen constantly and codeine at night seems to worsen the insomnia, as does the disco phrase now looping constantly inside my non-sleeping head. 'Feet don't fail me now!'

Simon is now prone to falling into The Hole. He's often silent. Moody. There's not much more he can take of everything going on, both in the Covid world outside and here inside our cancer world. Death is everywhere, the lockdown punishing, living as we all are a fully atomised, disconnected life, work disappearing, shrinking inside the boxes we live in, our colours fading, seeing no one, exacerbating the fear and the paranoia. Physically painful things are still happening to me and by extension to him. It's worse, I often think now, for the partners, driven to help at a fundamental level, and unable to. Even if they *do* help, merely by existing.

Kylie's latest disco-pop tickler 'Say Something' floats in from a radio, with lyrics which seem to relate to the endless pandemic. Can we, she wonders, in her Tinker Bell way, all be 'as one again?' Tears brim in my eyes.

To add plummeting hygiene standards to injury and insult, a lovely, refreshing, cleansing, piping-hot shower has become yesterday's dream-state luxury. For one month I'm banned from using the shower, the substantial mastectomy dressing unable to be soaked, wounds stubbornly refusing to heal. And it's summer. Washing my hair is now a lengthy palaver: kneeling on a pillow, wrapped in a towel by the side of the bath, leaning over the rim ladling water onto my head from a small saucepan filled blind from both cold and hot taps – freezing on one side, boiling on the other. A 'bath' is barely worth it, sitting in a six-inch puddle, towel around the neck and tucked under the right arm to shield the dressing. Apart from washing my legs and 'nethers' by just sitting there, I can slide a cloth all the way up and around my left arm, and my right arm up to the elbow. As with every other pleasure denied you 'in the process' of medical treatment, as soon as it's gone you're desperate to have it back, yearning for the blissful comforts of a sometime average day.

In late August, 'fresh' from a puddle bath, I whirl through the swanky, glass-fronted revolving front door of the central London hospital for radiotherapy pre-assessment, the hospital where the 'Clippity' Klopp lookalike embedded my excellent port. Once again, I realise my own ignorance: I know nothing about what radiotherapy entails, only grateful to be given it, marvelling once more at the thoroughness of what the NHS does for every individual.

A radiologist peers under the breast dressing and sees an open hole in one of the rows of stitches. I'm lying on my back so she helpfully takes a phone photo, to show me the circular flesh wound where a perky nipple once was – a photo I'm hoping she deletes immediately. Radiotherapy is delayed until November. They take body measurements anyway and ink a few tiny, permanent tattoo markers where lasers will meticulously line up, guiding a large rectangular blast of radiation through my reconstruction and onto the chest wall, incinerating any loitering, malicious cells.

Weekly check-ups with the surgeons follow, where they gingerly peel back the dressing to see the still-gaping hole where healed-up stitches should be. I've been using a prescribed ointment, expensive medical grade Manuka Honey, which is now deemed a miscalculation: it kept the wound site wet, and therefore open. 'I think we've been over-treating you!' they declare. The dressing is removed, a lighter one affixed 'to let the air in'. It works. All wounds dry up and heal, the dressing can come off at last.

And so, I see the breast reconstruction for the very first time, all the way round, in the full-length, living-room mirror.

It is horrendous.

This isn't a breast. Or anything like a breast. It's a dome of beige engineering stuck to the front of my body, swathed in my old, heavily scarred breast skin, a criss-cross pucker of stitches where a nipple once was. It bears no resemblance whatsoever to my remaining breast. I can see the base rim of the construction all the way round, like the rubber ring round the top of a condom, if worn by an elephant. Or a large rubber ball cut in half and superglued to my chest wall. It's solid, with the consistency of a medicine ball. I'm still grateful there's something there to fill the cavernous bra cup other than a sock, but it's a lot worse than any of the examples I was shown by the surgeon. It's disturbing because it's simply ... *inhuman*. Something alien is now grafted onto my otherwise human body. You can't look at it and not wince. No wonder the surgeon told me months ago patients' expectations are often 'too high'.

I would far rather have been shown the possible grim reality, or at least examples of the not-so-good alongside the can't-tell-which-one-is-fake. But it's understandable: this is difficult surgery, with countless variables depending on the individual. And if I'd been shown the example I'm currently staring at in the mirror I doubt I would have piped, in satisfaction, 'That's the very knocker for me!' By now I'd heard much anecdotal evidence that for some women a breast reconstruction, especially after a double mastectomy, is 'like a free boob job on the NHS!' Not this one, which I call my 'Mechanical Chest'. It also means I can't lie on my right side, my natural sleeping side, which also houses two ports; between these three foreign bodies embedded under my skin a good night's sleep is a long-faded memory. I can't imagine I'll ever sleep properly again. Obviously, since the start of all this back in autumn 2019, I have not aged a day. HEM HEM.

Perky Irish mum-pop troubadours the Nolan Sisters appear on breakfast TV. It's Linda and Anne, talking about their simultaneous recurring breast cancers, both with no hair. Linda now has secondary, incurable liver cancer. Pop reveller Sarah Harding from Girls Aloud, who I've interviewed many times, announces her stage four cancer diagnosis. She's been told she might not see another Christmas. I catch myself on. Sarah Harding is thirty-eight years old. A rubber ball where a breast once was, a wizened face and a fizzy, electrocuted foot, is nothing. No one has ever told me I have one year to live. I remain treatable. And may yet live to be fabulously ancient.

Unlike so very many of us.

25

CAN'T GET USED TO LOSING YOU

11 October 2017

It's my third *Smash Hits* funeral. First it was Tom 'Hibbs' Hibbert back in 2011, the man who sat next to me in my formative *Smash Hits* years, then deputy ed and the most brilliant comedic mind I'd ever encountered. At fifty-nine, he had gone off to the place he always called 'the hospital, for a very long time, i.e. for ever', to the tune of The Byrds' elevational dreamscape 'Eight Miles High'. Then it was Gavin Reeve-Daniels, the gifted *Smash Hits* designer-turned-nineties-ed, the assembled pinned to the pews as Simple Minds beseeched us all, 'Don't You (Forget About Me)'. Today, it's Richard Lowe, in his early fifties, the ed from '89 to '90, the scoundrel scouser who drank tea all day, each piping-hot mug accompanied by the quip he stole from a Rich Tea biscuit ad, as he sparked up another gasper, 'A drink's too wet without one' (which he would also say down the pub, as he lit an accompanying cig). An effortlessly cheeky chap, whenever my pre-pub ritual took place of applying lipstick in a hand-held mirror, he'd sidle up out of nowhere to announce three simple words: 'No hope, Sylv.'

Three of us from those *Smash Hits* days went to his funeral together: myself, lifelong pal and writer Tommy the D and another former *Smash Hits* ed, Mike Soutar (both fellow Scots).

Mike is by now an almost laughably successful publisher who'd singlehandedly pioneered the era of the magazine freesheet with *Shortlist* and *Stylist* magazines and is now known to millions as Lord Sugar's dastardly interviewing henchman on *The Apprentice*. He's known to me and Tom as Mike 'Soapy' Soutar, who we met when we were teenagers working for different teen titles at the DC Thomson publishing empire in Dundee. He was nicknamed, inevitably, after a character in Scotland's *Oor Wullie* cartoon, also published by DC Thomson, the annual of the spike-haired, dungareed, bucket-seated hero found in the Christmas stocking of every Scottish kid born from the 1940s onwards.

The ceremony itself was curiously religious with no overhead parps, as expected, from Richard's beloved Beatles. The congregation then headed to the wake where his wife Naomi, the sometime *Smash Hits* design ed, had organised wall-mounted screens showing pictures of the chirpy character we all remembered so well, usually wearing a fisherman's jumper, beloved cig always on the go. He'd been ill for some time, which is partly why we hadn't seen Richard for years: not since 2006, the year *Smash Hits* was banished to the layers of the cultural dumper. A classy, moving commemoration, it was also crushingly sad for Naomi and their grown-up daughter, and another mind-blowing reminder: we're losing our peers now, regularly, one by one.

Do we realise, that everyone we know someday will die? So sang Wayne Coyne, the frontman of masterfully poignant US mavericks The Flaming Lips, back in 2002, a then forty-year-old who knew, already, what was thundering towards him down rock's lost highway.

These days, especially after believing I was about to die, I think a lot about Spike Milligan, who I spent a night at the home of back in 1996. Then almost seventy-eight, he was very late for our interview, delayed at his doctor's, so suggested I stay in the spare room. His wife would give me a nightie, 'and we can have some cheese soldiers ... and some *wine*'. A man atomically built from mirth, a soliloquy he offered up that day has stayed with me ever since: 'I wake up every morning and think, Thank God, another day,' he twinkled. 'Every day I go out into a field and I lay down and I put a shovel by me and I wonder if anybody's going to bury me. And every day I come back and I say, "Guess what? I'm going to live!" Yes, ooh, this is very nice wine ...'

Where we're exceptionally good at comic genius in this country, we're exceptionally hopeless at death, which I confronted every day back in 2017 as the editor of a 'death positive' online start-up. Its mission was to engage the collective conscience with The Inevitable in a contemporary, digital way (an idea which ultimately failed; it was surely before its time). Talking to esteemed TV doctor Sarah Jarvis one day, she spelled out the problem: we've 'medicalised' death, hidden it away behind blue hospital curtains. Barely anyone dies at home any more, even if they want to; family members are woefully ill-equipped in every way to provide the necessary care. Conversations we need to have about end-of-life wishes are 'conversations we must have' but rarely do. It's the last taboo, the final too-frightening frontier. We live in a society where both vital scientific funding and mainstream media headlines concentrate overwhelmingly not on death, but on ways we can stay alive, for ever longer. This guarantees catastrophic consequences not only for the NHS, which uses vast resources in prolonging the life of the elderly whether there's quality of life or not, but for the already perilously over-populated planet itself.

Other cultures, I discovered that year, do death differently – better, more openly, realistically and significantly less squeamishly: coffins in Asia are proudly displayed on pavements outside coffin shops, Indonesian homes keep embalmed family members at home for months, Pacific islanders bury their parents in their gardens, Mexicans are much admired for their annual, skull-festooned carnival jamboree, the Day Of The Dead. Seeking original stories for the website, the subjects I commissioned included near-death experiences, losing a parent as a child, Alzheimer's, teenage suicide, and how it feels, as an adopted child, when the mother you never knew dies.

Over nine months, the spectre of death strode out of the shadows to take its rightful place in the light of everyday reality. I attended a Death Café, seated around a table with strangers talking about the deaths of loved ones (and who all laughed over how, as the saying goes, 'where there's a will, there's a writ'). A fascinating afternoon was spent with two Jewish-German Second World War refugees pouring over parchments and photos of their Holocaust memorabilia, almost all of their families having been murdered by the Nazis and so considering themselves 'the lucky ones'.

There were specialist freelance reports on how joyful hospices can be, a guide to helping a grieving friend, an interview with a woman planning to attend her own funeral aged seventy-four. After that, she chirped, 'the stupid gene kicks in', so would then take herself off to Dignitas. We ran an interview with a woman who'd lost her husband and best friend in a terrorist bombing, a review of an unfeasibly beautiful and ground-breaking exhibition on infant mortality, an interview with the best friend of a teenage victim of London's gang-related gun crime and a feature on 'comedy' funerals, starring rainbow-spray-painted hearses, celebrants dressed up as Darth Vader and flowers spelling out, instead of, say, 'GRANDAD', the word 'BASTARD'. It was not only one of the most absorbing jobs I've ever had but brought death, much more, into the centre of both my understanding and appreciation of life, where it belongs.

Death is coming to us all. We know it, and we must face it. And if we do, we become better at life, at nurturing relationships, at not wasting our finite time. If you're fortunate enough to reach your forties – and certainly by your fifties – the bodies *really* start piling up. In recent years, I've lost several old friends back in Scotland, who've all died relatively young – in their forties, fifties and early sixties. Rimmy is forever making gallows jokes about his social life revolving around funerals.

In 2022, more lights went out across the musical galaxy: fellow London bon viveurs through the nineties, Andy Ross (Food Records founder and the man who signed Blur, gone at sixty-five), Gavin Martin (music journalist and Belfast boy, at sixty), followed by Happy Mondays' Paul Ryder (Shaun's brother, hours before he was due on stage, at fifty-eight) and Foo Fighters' Taylor Hawkins (lost to tragically accidental folly, at fifty).

The historical contributors to the culture we love as kids also fire warning flares, whether the also recent deaths of the long-and-well-lived (grinsome gag-cannon Barry Cryer, eighty-six), or lives painfully cut short (early eighties' DJ figurehead Janice Long, sixty-six, a voice more familiar to me in the eighties than any member of my own family). And when Olivia Newton-John died from breast cancer in summer 2022, at seventy-three, I played her seventies' country songs and openly blubbed, singing along with that crystalline voice which originally made me love her, long before Bad Sandy in the leggings, with the fag.

But when death takes your peers, especially, it's a shocker every time. A ticking-clock jolt, a clanging reminder to get-busy-livin' which we all too easily forget, until the next time.

We will all attend the funerals not only of our families but all of our greatest friends, or they will attend ours (if they're not crocked in a care home by then). For all of us who reach mid-life, it's a permanent background noise, an audible foghorn on the looming horizon, over which so many have so suddenly disappeared. So, love them while they're here.

We are all just on loan to each other.

26

HELP THE AGED

I'm alive. I know that's all that matters. So why, when I look in the mirror and see my seventy-four-year-old mother on her deathbed staring back at me, does this bother me so much? It's not the getting old itself: on the contrary, for years I've held to the guiding maxim 'It is a *privilege* to grow old.' No. It's the looking old or rather, in my case, ten years older than I actually am. It's the crumbling, the corrosion, the disintegration into dust. I guess, therefore, it's because it looks so very close to death. But that's not what bothers so many of us across society today: we're acutely neurotic about looking old even when we're young. And often, *very* young.

It's partly conditioning, living in a culture which sees ageing as not only ugly, but outright grotesque, even a *failure* to somehow stay young. 'You look amazing!' congratulate the chat show hosts whenever yet another middle-aged millionaire with a twenty-five-year-old head as shiny as a newly glazed snooker ball dazzles on a TV sofa. It's a culture we not only encourage but personally invest in, financially, physically and emotionally, and increasingly so every year, even more so than in its industry subsidiary 'beauty'. The global anti-ageing market was worth an estimated $58.2 billion in 2020, while the global skincare market alone is estimated to reach a reported sparkly-eye-watering $189.3 billion by 2025.

The reason? The growing demographic shift – and exponentially so in the last twenty years – from middle-years consumers to the definitely still young.

Back in 2008, I interviewed alabaster, ginge-topped Girl Aloud Nicola Roberts who – after asking me my age, then forty-three – physically recoiled, exclaimed she was 'terrified' of ageing and wondered indeed aloud how I could stand it, how I coped? It was part of her job to be young and beautiful, but still, I was stunned: she was twenty-two at the time. Today, I doubt she'd feel the same, would give anything for her bandmate Sarah, gone at 39, and every one of those glorious Girls, including herself, to live to be *seriously* old.

But we don't think like that when we're young. I remember blurting out, at seventeen, when my mum wished me happy birthday, 'I feel past it already!' By twenty, I not only had a 'proper' job, but my Dream Job, staff writer on *Smash Hits*, and was too busy conducting misguided interviews with the likes of New Order's Bernard Sumner, then age thirty, and declaring him 'old' to his face, to ponder my own supposed decrepitude.

By thirty, I believed I *was* old, suddenly faced overnight with the perceived calamity of not-being-young any more, the close of my thirtieth birthday spent weeping on a night bus, alone, having been to see bubble-punk kitsch-kids Shampoo, distraught to think I still cared about children's music at this age, with less financial and emotional stability than I'd had at twenty-one. I'd newly joined the precarious freelance ranks of the *NME*, revelling along with Britpop's hedonistic hoopla, was single and living in a house share in Finsbury Park with two friends who were both about to leave to cohabit with their boyfriends (and in one case become a mum). I, on the other hand, was about to meet the man I believed was the love of my life, who turned out to be a wrong 'un, which left me bankrupt at thirty-three and hiding under a windowsill with the bailiffs banging on the door.

By forty, I was significantly more stable and optimistic, if still sporadically employed, holding a joint birthday party in London with sister Jackie, surrounded by my greatest London friends. Now in a relationship with Simon, it was eighteen months on from the death of my mother and I was about to buy my first (and almost certainly only) property while the magazine industry I'd worked in since aged eighteen was spiralling Down The Dumper.

By fifty, I was even less employed but bordering on euphoric while wandering the sun-drenched springtime streets of Paris – Simon's birthday present to me – the pair of us seated on vertical stone steps near the majestic Sacré Coeur, breaking off supermarket cheese and bread and pouring red wine into beakers from a delicious bottle of Beaujolais (three euros – a snip!)

All that time, though, through the decades to fifty, I'd never fixated on how old I looked, only how I *felt*. And through this fully subjective and non-scientific anecdotal evidence it seems to me – in the most ludicrous irony of all the contemporary neuroses – we worry much more about the concept of 'old', the younger we actually are.

No one wants to look decrepit, worn-out, fossil-faced and haggard. But you won't, with vigilance, decent food, hygiene, a bottle of water now and then, a good night's sleep and a power walk around the park. I have memories of interviewing incorrigible scouser and diva-pop force-of-nature Pete Burns in 2003, astounded at what the forty-three-year-old had done to his face in the name of youth and beauty: the peachy, line-free skin of a Girl's World prosthetic head, a taut, pink-glossed, lifebuoy ring where his lips once were and two parallel lines with ovals on the end where a handsome nose once was, the one he surely breathed through significantly more easily than he did through the one he now had.

'I'll be sitting in a restaurant,' he announced that day, in his winningly caustic way, puffing on a Marlboro Light, 'and some goon, some absolute *bricklayer* will stagger through the door and go, "Should I get my lips done or me penis enlarged?" I'm like, "Y'know, mate? I don't give a fuck if you have your arsehole enlarged." I'm not the boy next door. If you want the boy next door, fucking go next door.'

It was the kind of unapologetic belligerence we hadn't heard in contemporary pop since peak nineties' Oasis. He did what he did aesthetically, he carried on, with a single image in mind: 'Keith Richards: I cannot accept just looking at the same thing, decaying.'

Thirteen years later, in 2016, after extensive and continuous corrective surgeries on previously botched surgeries – because of which he developed blood clots in his legs, heart and lungs – the fabulously fur-coated Pete Burns died of a massive heart attack at the age of fifty-seven.

But by fifty-five myself I knew what he meant about decaying. I *obviously* was, through the intravenous poisons, the lack of nourishment, the lack of sleep and the cheek-caving weight loss. Today I'm Pete Burns' death-age – fifty-seven – fully nourished again, a stone heavier than I was in the Boney P months but the damage appears to be done. In the mirror I still see my mother's deathbed vision and *wince*. It feels, somehow, shameful. Like I should hide away in embarrassment. It *does* feel like I've failed, which makes me feel even more ashamed, because I know this isn't rational. It doesn't concern anyone else; not Simon, even though he's almost seven years younger than I am for a start, or my friends and family, not that they would mention it, not even brazen blabbermouth Ali. Because what's the alternative? It was either go through all that and come out the other side like *this*, or die. So I put my eyebrows on, delighted to even *have* eyebrows again, kick my own backside and rejoice in another day. Everything is in the attitude. And I've a better attitude now – so relieved, so *grateful* that I got to stay alive, when so many didn't – than I've ever had before.

The twenty-first century, meanwhile, is having none of it.

In 2022, Jeff Bezos, evidently bored by his toys-in-space already, announced his latest fantastical project, to Live For Ever, or at least extend the human lifespan by around fifty years. To this end, the fifty-eight-year-old man who wears sunglasses in the shape of love hearts, who is currently worth an estimated $188 billion (and every one of us who bought, say, a chopping board off Amazon because it was eight pounds cheaper than in Argos is to blame), announced he was backing new anti-ageing company Altos Labs, a biotech start-up which had newly announced three billion dollars in fresh funding. Within seconds he'd amassed a team of Big Pharma big-wigs, Nobel prize-winners and revered university professors reportedly being paid, 'sports-star salaries'. This is now the Holy Grail for idiot humanity that believes it can control everything – if it has enough money.

Every year we hear more reports of 'death-defying' science, the finest minds of a generation, alongside the richest and the most opportunistic, now collaborating on 'cellular programming', working on ways to eradicate diseases associated with growing old (heart disease, cancer, Alzheimer's), inventing drugs which flush away decaying cells, perfecting DNA-tampering techniques which will bring us a younger 'biological age'. None of which accounts for the fact that, if we do all live to be 150, the population of the planet will be approximately forty billion and counting and we'll have eaten the actual crust of the Earth itself, every other creature, plant and ecosystem surely gone, *scoffed*, for ever.

Or, even if the original, supposedly noble goal of eradicating disease comes to pass, these treatments will be available only for the wealthiest or hijacked for the cosmetic desires of the same wealthiest, or both. All of whom will then be living their biologically perfect lives with Bezos in a city-sized pod on Mars (while warfare over resources breaks out with Elon Musk's even bigger city-sized pod on Mars), while the rest of us ordinary, ugly, fatally diseased plebs perish on the barren, scorched Earth like rodents in a Californian wildfire.

On 8 January 2022, a Google homepage animation announced what would have been Stephen Hawking's eightieth birthday (shared with Elvis Presley, Dame Shirley Bassey and Dame David Bowie and therefore one of the greatest days in the calendar to be born). Created by Google's art lead, Matthew Cruickshank, the two minute 'Google Doodle' was worked on and approved by the Hawking family, the voice of the celebrated boffin generated to create a speech made up of some of his best-loved quotes. The message, excerpted here, was characteristically enlightening, one we'd all do well to heed over the billionaires currently attempting to defy life's only true inevitable (where we used to say 'death and taxes', the taxes bit no longer, to them, applies). And who, in their quest to eradicate imperfection, might one day also bother to eradicate motor neurone disease, and if that had happened eighty years ago would've meant a standard life for the esteemed professor, possibly to the detriment of scientific theory and cosmological understanding today. Where we'd all rather see an end to this dreadful, cruel disease, it's still a thought. Swings and roundabouts.

My name is Stephen Hawking. My expectations were reduced to zero at twenty-one. Everything since then has been a bonus. Although I cannot move and have to speak through a computer, in my mind I am free ...
    One of basic rules of the universe is that nothing is perfect. Perfection simply doesn't exist. Without imperfection neither you nor I would exist ... However bad life may seem, where

there is life, there is hope. Be brave. Be curious. Be determined. Overcome the odds. It can be done.

If only I'd heard that message the day I was confronted with a psychological test I definitely didn't see coming. One I could not overcome.

27

WEAK AS I AM

July 2020 in Sad Kitchen and I'm not feeling sad at all. I'm four cans of cider in, which has taken several hours to sip through, the first night I've been drinking properly after six months of no alcohol whatsoever. Simon's gone to bed and transcendental sixties' Bee Gees music wafts, harmoniously, from Alexa.

It starts with some sort of brain twinge. A synapse, surely, has twitched, igniting a spark of memory, some dormant region of the hippocampus firing back into life. Something is telling me, as Richard Lowe from *Smash Hits* always used to say: a drink's too wet without one. Six months have passed since I banished my vape to the back of the kitchen-table drawer, supposedly for ever, and the sneaky addict within has made a wholly unexpected comeback, barging unstoppably into my psyche and convincing me I'm desperate for the other half of the perfect Friday night combination (as Oasis always knew): cigarettes and alcohol.

Just for the one night, I think, as all addicts always do. The second I think that thought I know there's no going back. Now I can physically feel an acceleration of the chemical changes in my brain, a tingling under the scalp, the well-worn neurological pathways of historical addiction crackling back into life, four pints of cider all the jump leads it evidently needs. Nicotine addiction, like all true addictions, is an insidious Frankenstein's monster and I have wilfully switched on the power.

All my life I've been afraid of addiction, as kids of alcoholics so often are. Some react by leading a teetotal life, which was never the case for me: if anything, it was the opposite, barrelling through my youth in hedonistic abandon, jubilant on the outside, fearful on the inside that the alcoholism baton had been passed to me, as it had been passed to my mother by her draconian, abusive father (who eventually took his own life). But I always felt, at least *hoped*, it would be me who stopped the cycle.

As a young booze enthusiast I could be prone to emotional chaos, to blackouts, to bouts of weeping, of never knowing when to stop (thankfully, no more) but I also knew I wasn't, as she was, a volatile Jekyll and Hyde, someone who so clearly metamorphosed into a dramatically frightening stranger. Her alcoholism was abruptly guillotined only by prison, an outrageously harsh experience for a sixty-three-year-old widow, incarcerated for three months in 1995 for the crime of persistently calling the ambulance service in a cry for help (and then punching a paramedic). Post-prison, she was finally sober if psychologically fragile for the rest of her life, left with the addiction that led to her death from the lung condition COPD: smoking.

Over the decades I've talked to scores of public figures, maybe hundreds, who've wrangled with addictions – mostly alcohol and drugs – and listened to their stories of spiralling dependence, of squalid rock bottom, of enlightenment and recovery. Conversations which taught me, among much else, how much my mum needed empathy and professional help so much more than criminalisation and imprisonment.

I've talked several times to Britain's sometime No. 1 Celebrity Rock'n'Roll Drug Addict, Pete Doherty, and found him both a gentle, cerebral soul and dangerously lost to the tyrannical overlord of addiction. The first time was 2007, then on a methadone programme during a brief pause from heroin. We sat together on his unkempt, purple duvet-topped bed, in the small bedroom of his East End Hackney flat, its front door boarded up, a student bombsite strewn with old and bloodied needles, with two late-teenage female fans barefoot on his sofa. His famed 'blood paintings' were daubed on the walls, daubings indeed; one brown stain with a vague approximation of the number seven was supposedly a portrait of George Best. With enormous, baleful brown eyes, his mouth was permanently open, a blister on his bottom lip crusted over in black, with the matching sooty fingers of a Dickensian child up a chimney. Softly spoken to the point of inaudible, he cut a harmless jib, buoyed by the soporific flow of the watery, methadone dream-state. After ten minutes of conversational chaos (he kept breaking into caterwauling song), he threw his crack pipe on the bed. It was fashioned from a miniature bottle of Bailey's Irish Cream, sawn off at the bottom with a black filter inside the neck, the reason his fingers and bottom lip were black. He mumbled something I couldn't hear which made me respond, 'But that's like saying you don't care about yourself, that's no good.'

'Even my dad won't talk to me,' he replied. 'He thinks I'm a disgrace. He says, "You're not my son."'

He fiddled with two crumpled wraps, lodged a small white rock the size of a matchstick tip onto the black filter, filled his whole mouth with the bottom of the bottle, lit and inhaled the smoke curling around inside, a particularly dense grey bringing to mind a nineteenth-century tuberculosis ward. It was not only the first time I'd witnessed a musician smoke crack during an interview; it was the first time I'd ever seen *anyone* smoke crack. There was now nothing to be done except sit in silence watching Pete Doherty's closed eyes, both eyeballs clearly moving behind those enormous lids, from side to side, side to side, in synchronised slow motion until the wave had finally passed.

'What's happened to your methadone programme?'

'This is just weed.'

'Oh, this is ridiculous . . . they look like rocks to me, mate.'

He laughed and proffered a fist-bump. He felt he was clean, evidently, because this wasn't heroin – crack didn't count.

I persevered. 'Some of the people who come round this flat are kids. But you're a twenty-seven-year-old adult now.'

'Well, it's not simple, addiction. I never wanted to be a role model and I don't wanna encourage it. I don't.'

'Other people think you're squandering your talent, but do you think you are?'

'No . . . no . . . no . . . no. I don't know what I'm doing.'

'Is this the rock'n'roll dream?'

'It's *a* dream.' He flicked his lighter. 'I don't know how all this happened. How it got like this. I'm just a little schmindie songwriter. Yeah, man. That's it. And I'm bringing the good name of schmind down. With all this. Whatever happened to just sitting in a graveyard dressed in black?'

Seven years later, in 2013, the now thirty-four-year-old Pete Doherty was seated at a wooden table outside the Lord Stanley pub near Camden, north London, two years on from the death of his friend (and, briefly, lover) Amy Winehouse, who'd lived a few streets away from here. Now living in Paris, escaping the British tabloids, he was emotional that day, tearful, over Amy and other friends who'd died, but was far more lucid, off the crack, drinking Sailor Jerry spiced rum and analysing the nature of addiction. I'd brought along addiction scholar Russell Brand's 2011 eulogy to Winehouse and we read it together.

'Addiction is a serious disease,' wrote Brand, on his website. 'It will end with jail, mental institution or death. Not all addicts have Amy's incredible talent. Or Kurt's or Jimi's or Janis's, some people just get the affliction. All we can do is adapt the way we view this condition, not as a crime or a romantic affectation but as a disease that will kill. We need to review the way society treats addicts; not as criminals but as sick people in need of care.'

'That's what people thought originally, when heroin was pharmaceutically created,' mused Pete. 'But it's seen as a spiritual crime now, to be a junkie, the lowest thing.'

His emotions resurfaced, tearfully describing the zero tolerance letters he received in prison from Second World War vets telling him the freedom they fought for allowed 'a disgrace' like him to flourish.

'What do you see addiction as?'

'I see it as a selfish lifestyle choice,' he replied, evidently not seeking any sympathy. 'My nine-year-old son. I can't be there for him.'

Recently, he'd taken his son Astile through Spain on tour. Did he ask questions about drugs?

'Yeah, he's smart. He said to me, "Have you just taken your medicine?" I didn't know what to say. In his eyes it's sad and wrong, you're not the attractive person a child wants you to be.'

'Russell Brand also wrote that all addicts are "not quite present" when you talk to them.'

'Not quite as present as who, though?' he frowned, before a curiously detached rumination on the necessity of detachment, perhaps long resigned that he can't really be there for anyone. 'If there's someone who you've let down or shamed or alienated, who doesn't feel that you're there – whether it's your father, son, friend – you will just remove yourself from them,' he coolly explained of the addict's mindset. 'The sad fact is, that's what destroys families, because you separate and surround yourself with people who will let you believe you're still a whole person. Because who wants to admit those things? Who wants to admit that's who they are?'

'You've said before you'll only change if you hit "rock bottom". Are you anywhere near?'

'Not right this second, no. But I'm ultra-skilled in manipulating my own feelings. I've had to be. This is my life.'

It would be six more years until forty-year-old Pete Doherty, in 2019, was finally on the road to freedom from crack and heroin – and all it took was a combination of a double arrest in Paris over forty-eight hours, pissing all over the reception counter of a Parisian police station, conditional probation forcing him to take a heroin-blocking injection called Buvidal and a dealer-isolating global pandemic. Addiction: it's a serious disease, all right.

Opening the kitchen-table drawer in Sad Kitchen in 2021, there they are, two of them, small, almost-diamond shaped, nestled amongst the metal coils, bottles of juice (mixed fruit) and battery chargers. I'm giving in to my selfish lifestyle choice. These are not Pete Doherty's crack pipes, there's nothing here that will kill me or put me in prison or a mental institution, but they're full of a drug I've long 'kicked', a drug which compromises my life, which has made me ill for ever, which I'm wilfully welcoming back tonight in the year health has never felt more precious.

Picking up my most recent vape, for the first time in six months, it's still half full of juice. Placing the plastic rim to my lips, I deeply inhale . . . and nothing. Out of battery of course. *Damn it.* A sense of panic, but I can fix it and call on reserves of patience. I plug the battery in, it's working!

Twenty minutes later I'm inhaling again . . . and nothing. The vape itself is simply not working. *Bollocks.* But that's OK because I have the other one! The inner addict smiles, sneakily, knowing exactly why she merely threw that vape in the back of the drawer, alongside the other old one and didn't throw them *out.* Because, y'know, just in case. Exactly the same thing happens again. Inhale, nothing, charge, wait, nothing. Also broken. *Bastards.* Hot anger flushes across my cheeks.

I think there might be another one, a really old one . . .

Rummaging further in the drawer . . . it's there! The seven-year-old vape which, in comparison to the modern designs, is the size and shape of a clarinet. I puff on that, too, vigorously. *Nothing.* I attempt to charge that one and . . . more nothing. Battery dead, vape dead, *you lose.* There's nothing I can do. No alternative whatsoever. Not like in the olden days as a teenager when I'd sprinkle tea leaves into torn-out pages of a Bible kept around the house, the paper as delicate as Rizlas, roll it up and attempt to smoke it, with inevitable fringe-singeing results.

I stare at the surface of the too-big Vincent van Gogh table, now a graveyard of vaper's paraphernalia, and think: *You sad bastard.* You don't need it. You've already *proved* you don't need it. I shunt everything back in the drawer and step away from the table, glad Simon isn't here to witness this woeful weakness, after all this time. My brain stops sparking, I can feel it giving up, the voice of the sneaky addict within simply shuts up. And I go to bed.

The following morning I'm so relieved I'm ecstatic. They didn't work! Man, that was close. This time, I take all the paraphernalia out of the drawer, walk to the communal bins outside the block and throw everything away. This time, finally, it's over.

It's still over. Since 20 January 2020 I have not smoked a thing. *Nothing whatsoever.* I tried, just that once, but I couldn't and therefore I haven't. I can't remember the last time I coughed. I can't believe, now, there were times of heavy smoking when I could barely breathe at all; at best like breathing through a straw in my neck, terrifying incidences of constricted airways, out of nowhere, walking along the street in daylight. The freedom of not thinking about smoking any more is one of the greatest liberties I've ever known.

When you're a smoker, today, there are always restrictions in public, so you're for ever wondering where and when your next fagging opportunity will arise. It never leaves your mind. Serious addiction is stronger than any one person's will. I'm pleased for the young today that nicotine, generally, isn't a big one for them (they have The Phones to deal with instead). I know no young people who are regular smokers. Maybe the odd 'sneaky' on a night out. I have my suspicions about weed (with, given my history, absolutely no leg to stand on).

Culturally, thankfully, we're in a different era now. No young person ever sits in smoke-filled offices as I did in the eighties and nineties, ashtrays spilling over every desk, or in smoke-hazed pubs and clubs. It's all over for the Reaper's once-dominant killer, overtaken by the spectrum of killer mental health issues instead.

Another unexpected benefit, as equally life-enhancing, is the return of the full-effect taste bud. It's taken a while but since mid-2021 – well over a year post-vape and the last of the Mouth Hell – food has never tasted this delicious, *ever*. Everything, as soon as it hits the tip of my tongue, is an explosion of sensory pleasure. 'Hmm-hmmmmm!' is now a daily yelp, from explosively flavoursome chilli to the sweetness of a simple apple. I'd been living a savour-free half-life for decades and didn't even know it. 'It's the little things,' we're always told and it's the little things and no mistake. The little things are unquestionably the biggest things of all, the nourishing things, be they food, family, nature, culture, friendship, or a rollicking good laugh with anyone you love at the silliness of it all.

Today, for the very first time in my life, I don't think it, I *know* it: I'll never smoke anything ever again. After forty years I'm not only no longer addicted to nicotine, I don't *care* about nicotine any more. Never think about it. No matter how many pints of cider. I'm not addicted, in fact, to *anything* any more. I'm not my mother. I'm free. It's one of the greatest gifts cancer has given me.

28

RADIO GA GA

Radiotherapy treatment is like being abducted by aliens. I'd imagine. Padding into a huge, white, windowless room, wearing the hospital gown, I arrive on the deck of the Starship *Enterprise*. Large rectangular screens hang down from the ceiling, on which rows of numbers sit, as baffling to me as ancient hieroglyphics. My name, date of birth and first line of address are also on the screen, which I'm asked to confirm. Swinging onto a treatment bed, strangers' hands shunt my torso up, down, sideways. It's a busy room, with four young radiologists at work, one of whom folds down my gown so my deviant breast is inches away from their faces. Their work begins, information exchanged and verified.

'Nine-point-seven ... nine-point-five ... lovely coverage ... good on the top ...'

They disappear, press buttons in the adjacent viewing room and expansive wings of machinery slide up from the floor in a circular motion, soon positioned overhead. Only now can you see the stickers affixed to the underside of the machine: dolphins, unicorns, sparkles, a comedy turtle, cats with love-heart eyes. Kids, of course (and their parents) deal with this every day. Neon green laser beams shoot out from unidentified sources and line up with the tattooed dots penned two months ago. I can see inside the hood of the machine, through a small glass window, where two horizontal metal 'doors' with comb-like teeth move towards each other, programmed to open and close depending on where the radiation needs to beam. They have to make sure, I'm told one day, the radiation doesn't leak out a micro-millimetre – into, say, the lungs. Aiiiieeeee! This is why, they add, there's a slight possibility that radiotherapy could *cause* cancer in the future.

'It's all about making sure nothing comes back,' a friendly radiologist tells me. '*Trying* to make sure. It really is an excellent treatment.'

Radiotherapy works a lot like chemo, targeting sinister cells, only this time from the outside in, over a specific area of the body. As the surgeon said some months ago, I need this as well as the mastectomy, 'because I can't be certain I get every cell'.

It's the DNA within every cell which controls how it grows and divides, and radiation is targeted to damage DNA, causing the whole cell to eventually die, within weeks. Radiation will also damage healthy cells, causing tolerable side effects (burning skin, itching, swelling, tissue damage, the aforementioned infinitesimal chance of causing cancer), but at first it kills cells which are actively dividing, which cancer cells do far faster than healthy cells (of course they do, the clever bastards). A standard three-week course of almost daily radiotherapy is usually enough to see the alien cells exterminated.

In the radiotherapy room, music pipes gently overhead, which makes me think, once again, how in public you rarely hear the Music of Now, it's always the Music of Then. Over the coming weeks I'll be lulled here on the table by Chic's 'We Are Family', Air Supply's 'I'm All Out of Love', Crowded House's 'Always Take The Weather With You' and (the universe having a laugh once more) Roy Orbison's 'Pretty Woman'.

Every day I walk around five kilometres through the damp and chill of a London late autumn while the skin on my reconstruction and surrounding chest wall turns an itchy, burnished copper. My threadbare hair, bald at the sides, thin on top, is slowly growing back, the new hair at the crown sprouting like Rod Stewart's in the 1970s, all wiry, coarse and manly.

One day in the radiotherapy clinic waiting room, a nearby young couple in their thirties are colouring in a book with their little boy, around four years old, who has no hair whatsoever. A nurse approaches to greet them (there's a special waiting area here for kids).

'D'you wanna come to the playroom, Ben?'

Ben: 'Yaaaaaay!'

In the waiting room alongside us, fifteen people of various ages, from twenty-somethings to seventy-somethings, spontaneously burst into applause. It's our way of saying, I guess, 'I'm really sorry, lovely young couple ... and please, universe, spare this little chap.' What Ben would do, I think to myself, for a sprig of my Rod Stewart hair?

For three weeks, every weekday, all I do is walk towards public transport, sit on public transport, walk some more, head into hospital, walk back towards public transport, walk home. Not for the first time I think, how can people with proper jobs *do* this? One answer, of course, is sick pay. During one sixteen-minute wait at Finsbury Park overground, I'm walking up and down the platform, partly to keep warm, partly to get my steps in, using these daily hospital visits to at least complete an invigorating walk. It's very cold, my eyes are streaming, so I'm sporadically dabbing at leaky eyes. Striding back from the platform's end, on the way to the other end, a Transport For London staffer in a hi-vis jacket approaches.

'Excuse me, are you all right?'

'Sorry?'

(Leaning into my face) 'Are you *all right?*'

(Penny dropping) 'Oh! Oh yes, thank you, I'm absolutely fine!'

'Are you *sure* you're all right?'

'I'm sure, I'm just getting my steps in! And I've got streamy eyes.'

'Well, if you're sure you're all right ...'

Bless Transport For London. It's staffers like these who've either seen with their own eyes, or dealt with the aftermath of, human beings throwing themselves in front of oncoming trains from the exact spots where I've been persistently wafting a man-size Kleenex. It's both a comforting and conflicted thought, that here in the bedlam of the capital, where so many troubled souls will perish, there are strangers among us looking out for other strangers, even if it's tragically part of their job: so many souls, year after year, staring at locomotives thundering down tracks with a fathomless despair this lightly burnished radiotherapy patient has never known and can only hope never will.

The Amy book has been handed in, a book which more than compounds my thoughts on contemporary fame through the recollections of her lifelong best friend. Tyler emphasised many times how much he blamed fame for her death and for months I'd listened to the case for the prosecution: how fame imprisoned her, skewed her reality, left her ridiculed, belittled, riven with insecurity. I'd seen it personally back in 2006 when we spent two days together in New York, Amy a self-harming, image-paranoid bulimic even before her rekindled romance with Blake, who introduced her to the world's worst drugs. She'd never heard of the magazine I was from, the mighty and much-missed *The Word*. 'Is it British or American?' she wondered at the photoshoot that day, fretting that her self-applied makeup was a mess. 'British? That's OK, they already know I'm ugly.'

Fame destroyed her already fragile self-esteem, loosened her already tenuous grip on trust, and she became increasingly bedevilled by extreme bulimia and violent self-harm. In the last three years of her life, she was finally drug-free and trapped inside her home, now a binge-drinking alcoholic, the paparazzi living in cars outside her front door. She felt cut off from both friendship and society, fame warping how everyone treated her, as something other than a normal person, becoming lonelier and lonelier, with Tyler her lone companion, her other housemates her twenty-four-hour monitoring bodyguards. In the last few weeks of her life she'd continually say she was tired. 'I just don't want this life, Tyler,' she told him. 'Would you ever wanna be famous, really? I hate it. I'm bored of it. And I'm tired.' It was like, he openly wept one day, she was tired of life. At twenty-seven years old.

Understandably, Tyler can't bring himself to read the book for some weeks. While I wait, work enters an impasse: there isn't any, Christmas is approaching, so I 'spring'-clean the flat, obsessively, a way to feel productive. I'm still cleaning every day two weeks later and feel like Amy Winehouse having one of her crack-fuelled, OCD, clean freak episodes (she had many of those). With no cleaning duties left, I paint our sorry hallway, water damaged the year before by the leaky roof. I'm now the kind of person who excitedly buys Stain Block at the local hardware store, strides home purposefully, sprays it all over the corner of the hallway, stands back and marvels as if witnessing one of Turner's finest in the National Gallery. DIY completed, I'm then watching a vintage *Star Trek* boxset, the first TV series I ever fell in love with, starring my first-ever TV romantic crush, the twinkle-eyed interplanetary crumpeteer Captain James T. Kirk.

My treatment plan, meanwhile, is morphing again: towards Christmas all I'll have is the Kadcyla treatment every three weeks, the tolerable, targeted new chemo, until the following summer, which means I'll edge, incrementally, back towards normality. Or this new normality, at least, the Covid-restricted one we've all been living in (with the notable exception of the rule-setting UK government). By November's end this unrelenting fandango will have taken up a year of my life, a year where I've tramped through every season, around parks and streets, now into my second winter of life defined by illness, in a *world* defined by illness. And then, on 2 December, breaking news ... science has released a vaccine. It's called Pfizer. It *works*. This thing is coming to an end! Isn't it?

Not quite. Soon, London is under 'Tier 4' Covid restrictions, so our broken-down kitchen becomes our new favourite pub, not that we've any choice. Simon fetches the lamp from the hospital side-room days, sits it beside the first lamp he ever bought me back in 2005, when I was pregnant, something he bought for the 'bairn's room', even though we didn't have a bairn's room and shortly after no bairn either. Today, he grandly names the pub, The Two Lamps. We even make a paper sign for it and Sellotape it to the kitchen door whenever the pub is open. Which is quite a lot. It's now unfathomable to me how I managed to not drink for six months, considering how much of a stress-buster these nights in the Lamps have proved to be.

21 December 2020.

Simon's forty-ninth birthday, the 'shortest day' of the year, so technically the worst day in the calendar to have a birthday. 'It's true!' he hollers, adding it's impossible to have a proper party, 'because people are usually travelling, stressed out or gone home for Christmas already.' Over the years, in what is now a tradition, something unforeseen has gone wrong on his birthday, as if to prove his point – freak snow, cancelled tubes and buses, emergency dental surgery, pulled muscles, burned pizzas, even going to the pictures to see a 'classic' film that was so boring we walked out halfway through. This year we've no options, perhaps thankfully. We can only go for a walk and come home to The Two Lamps, where we order a takeaway from our favourite local Indian.

Simon: 'Hello. Can I order a delivery please?'

Takeaway dude: 'Um … um … I'm sorry, sir, could you ring back again in maybe five minutes?'

Simon: 'Oh? Sorry, are you really busy?'

Takeaway dude: 'No, it's our chef, he's just fainted.'

Simon: 'He's *what?*'

Takeaway dude: 'Just two seconds ago. He's currently unconscious on the kitchen floor.'

Simon: 'Oh! Well, I … um … I hope he's all right? OK. Well … thanks …'

He hangs up.

'See? It's my birthday!'

Twenty-third of December marks my second Christmas week in the chemo suite, where Prince the nurse has now been promoted and newbie staff are marvelling, all over again, at my 'beautiful!' port. The winter wave of Covid infection is here, my forthcoming bone density scan cancelled as the hospital fills with the Covid-struck once more. The rest of Europe and the *New York Times* are now referring to the UK as 'Plague Island'. Everyone has had enough. I see a TV ad featuring Chris Rea's 'Driving Home For Christmas' as the flashbacks arrive of the MRI scan and the wonky headphones and the breasts drooped in plastic moulds, as if to drive home the one-year anniversary. After months of thinking I'll never be irritated or sad or angry about anything ever again, I realise I've been all those things in recent weeks, and consciously remind myself that all that matters is staying alive and the people you love.

Christmas Day 2020.

Like most of the UK (and beyond) we spend Christmas in lockdown, at home. Late morning we head out to a bench in

Alexandra Park, with a couple of cans, Stella for him, Strongbow for the 'lady'. Parked on the bench like bums in the winter sun, it's one of the best Christmas mornings ever. The next-along bench has the same idea, two middle-aged women (and possibly very middle-class) popping an actual bottle of champagne. A robin flies out of the tree in front of us and lands near our bench, bouncing around our feet. Our very own Christmas robin: what could be better? (Clue: the fact Simon does not make any space cakes this year and keeps true to his vow that he never will again.)

January 2021 dawns and the world is still in lockdown. We do a Hogmanay Zoom quiz with Trish, Gilly B and their partners and wait for the madness to stop. It doesn't stop. The chemo suite was moved again as the winter Covid surge arrived and is now in the oldest part of the hospital, a long-disused maternity ward hastily reconfigured to house chemo patients as far away from the Covid-bedevilled main wards as possible. By early 2021 I breeze into this third chemo suite like the veteran patient I now am.

'All right Prince?'

'Morning Sylvia! Take a seat.'

'Morning Nadia! Morning Bimpe!'

I've seen these people significantly more than I've seen my own family and friends in Scotland since May 2019, almost two years, in an environment more familiar to me than any pub with my London pals in the last twelve months. Settling into the reclining seat, looking up beyond the blue curtain, a single string of white fairy lights Sellotaped onto the ceiling do their very best to bring festive cheer as the poisonings all around begin. Today, after two weeks of postponed treatment due to low red blood cells, my Kadcyla dose has been reduced. My body, Prince tells me, 'will be feeling pretty beaten up by now'.

The final body blows, though, are still to come.

29

(NOT) LOVING THE ALIEN

Seventeen months on from first discovering a dodgy nipple, I look down at my Mechanical Chest in the shower in early February 2021 and think, once again: what the hell is THAT? The implant is glowing red, burning hot to the touch, bigger than usual, even more solid than usual. I've not been feeling well, still working through the Kadcyla treatments, have chills and feel feverish again although the thermometer says I'm OK.

Two days pass and the Mechanical Chest begins to slowly blow up, as if affixed to a bicycle pump. On the third day, it pumps up some more, into the monstrous shape of a gigantic, crimson octopus head. Texting nurse Renée, she tells me to go, immediately, to A&E.

Within the hour I'm once again in an episode of *24 Hours in A&E*, waiting in a plastic armchair in a corridor while harassed young staff bustle at speed, logging people in. A young, tearful mother carries her eighteen-month-old son in her arms and explains he's swallowed a penny.

Eventually, I'm escorted to a side room where a nurse performs obs before a young male doctor arrives. 'That's definitely not right,' he concludes, coolly observing my topless torso, half of which now resembles a scarlet space hopper from the 1970s, without the amusing face. He disappears and surgical assistant Martha, suddenly, is there.

This is what the reconstruction leaflets warned me about: a 'seroma', a collection of fluid within the engineered breast – blood, possibly poisonous infection – which must be drained. The overlying skin is now as taught as a timpani and *bloody sore*, an emergency ultrasound hastily booked.

Lying on yet another table, staring upwards at yet more grey-white ceiling panels, the sonographer squirts gel around the radioactive space hopper, traces the ultrasound around the mound and locates the fluid on his screen. 'Sharp scratch,' comes the warning I've now heard a thousand times, as yet another harpoon looms into view, a thick, lengthy, hollow needle attached to a whopping empty syringe, soon filling up with hot, deep-red blood. I watch, as if hypnotised by a horror movie, as the Mechanical Chest begins to deflate directly under my chin, collapsing in on itself like a violently punctured beach ball, ridges appearing and folding towards each other. One giant syringe is filled, then another one, then half of another one. The relief – of the heat, the tightness, the pressure – is immense. Even if I'm left with what now appears to be a *half-eaten* octopus head glued to the front of my body.

Within days, it fills up again. And so I'm harpooned again.

Two weeks later it fills up again. I'm harpooned again.

On 20 April 2021, one year on from the constipation debacle (and still Hitler's birthday), the after-effect of the harpooning episodes is so painful it's like I've had the mastectomy all over again. I must return to painkillers I'm loath to take (still not touching the morphine). Admin chores also must carry on regardless, delicately padding to the local chemist to pick up the next batch of my five-year prescription for Letrozole, the oestrogen-diminishing drug which helps keep cancer cells at bay while turning me into even more of a geezer than I now definitely am, what with the one real bosom and the Rod Stewart hair.

Ali rings for a catch-up and a nosebleed begins in the street, gushing into the top of my Covid mask. Darting up a side street, I whisk the mask off and attempt to stem the flow with a hanky, while her voice carries on. 'Are you all right? What's happened!?' Up a side road by a taxi rank, my hand pinched over the top of my nose with blood streaks down to my chin, I look like the latest victim of a London stabbing, albeit fortunately (compared to most) in the face.

Two weeks later, the Mechanical Chest blows up again, so I'm harpooned again. And two weeks later, again. One week later, again and this time, staggeringly, the pain is even worse. We're now into May. This particular episode of the pain process has been going on since February and the pain within the mechanism itself is now so bad it hurts when I *breathe in*, never mind lie down, move in bed, get up, sneeze or – very occasionally – laugh. I've had no sleep whatsoever for many nights and have had to give up home yoga, something I'd discovered alongside millions of others in lockdown, via *Yoga with Adriane* online, which makes me feel taller and more balanced and stretchier and generally better. And now that's been taken away, too. Turning to Google, I learn of something called capsular contracture from breastcancer.org.

Once a breast implant is in place, fibrous scar tissue forms around it, creating a tissue capsule. The body forms a protective capsule like this around any object it recognises as foreign. The tissue capsule is usually soft or slightly firm, not noticeable, and helps to keep the implant in place. In some women, a tissue capsule forms that is unusually hard and dense. The capsule tightens around and squeezes the implant. This condition, called capsular contracture, can cause chronic pain and distortion in the shape of the breast, and it can make the breast rise higher on the chest. If you've had radiation therapy at any time in the past – and particularly if you had it after your initial breast reconstruction surgery – that can greatly increase your risk of developing capsular contracture.

Blinking at the words, I know I'm a textbook case. Something no one has mentioned. It's fixed either through corrective surgery or removing the implant and creating a new breast 'flap' from a fleshy part of your body or just removing The Monster and living with a heavily scarred chest wall. As seventies' glam-pop hobos The Sweet once said, I haven't got a clue *what* to do. Ms Jana finds a window to see me, prescribes three types of painkiller, which will definitely cause constipation (but now I *always* own a family-sized box of laxative sachets), and makes another appointment for another harpooning. 'It might just work this time.' She also prescribes industrial-strength antibiotics for twelve days. I mention capsular contracture and she agrees it could be that, exacerbated by radiotherapy, but let's deal with the seroma first.

This week the Mechanical Chest is so hard, mounded and high up, it looks a giant, flesh-coloured Tunnock's Teacake stuck to my body. The other one, meanwhile, with the weight loss, looks like an oven glove. *Anything* will be better than this.

The next ultrasound is performed by a heavy-handed sonographer who presses so hard I'm being pummelled in the uppermost ribs. She's being thorough, locating only tiny pockets of fluid, not enough for the needle to extract. There's no seroma left. 'There's nothing we can do,' she announces, the first time anyone in the NHS has ever said those words to my face. It makes me think about all the terminally ill people across the planet who hear that most-dreaded phrase every day. And so, once again, even as I lie bare-chested and broken on this surgical bed, staring up at the '3 a.m. Eternal' ceiling, I feel a deep acknowledgement of my personal ongoing luck.

Back in the consultation room, Ms Jana declares the

reconstruction 'failed'. My body is 'hyper-sensitive' and the implant must be removed.

Hyper-sensitive. I've had enough of being hyper-sensitive! Why can't I be the hardest woman in Britain!?

It's a lot to take in, once again. I don't even know what it means: will I be stitched up with half a flat torso for ever? Will there be an alternative implant solution in the future? And what happens to all the dangling skin left over?!

Ms Jana explains I can have the 'flap' reconstruction later, officially known as a DIEP flap, where skin, fat and blood vessels are sliced (usually) from your lower abdomen and used to fashion a new breast. DIEP stands for the 'deep inferior epigastric perforator' blood vessels which run through the abdomen and sound, frankly, like something your body can't do without. However, with the weight loss I'm not 'fleshy' enough yet for a flap but if I want it in a fleshier future, I can have it. Right now, I'm not concerned with the future, I just want The Monster gone and to be free from persistent pain.

At home I become the kind of person who googles mastectomy bras. They are very nice, lacy and womanly, with little pockets you place the 'breast form' in. For the first time it sinks in like a plummeting stone down a well: I'm about to be a one-knockered woman. Finally, this disturbs me. It's not even about being womanly, or not, it's about being ... mutilated. It's an amputation. The thought of what this will look like – sad, ludicrous, definitely grotesque – is a debilitating negative to feel about your own body, a body I've been reasonably at peace with throughout all the physical fluctuations of life, at least relative to the extreme neuroses which dominate society today. The thought of Simon seeing my naked upper body is even worse (I'd spared him the implant horrors, never taking off my bra): he's squeamish, can't look at surgery on TV, he'll wince at best, never want to touch me there again at worst.

It's just not possible, I'm certain, to feel or be thought of as attractive, naked, ever again. But I also know being dead is significantly *less* attractive. And then *again*, he has a club foot and it's never stopped me enthusiastically leaping on. So all I have to do is conjure up perspective and images of the Paralympians and I'm ready for The Monster to be slain.

30

TAKE ME OUT

Another 7 a.m. hospital check-in, on a balmy, late May morning, 2021. In an unknown Northern ward, another lifetime first: fondling a pair of disposable knickers, which were waiting for me on the bed. Their simplicity is perplexing, a very loosely elasticated piece of fragile gauze with fraying edges where the legs go in. Also waiting are a pair of anti-embolism socks to thwart deadly blood clots.

A nurse asks many questions, including the hitherto preposterous, 'Do you have carers at home?' I'm given two paracetamol, one ibuprofen and a visit from Ms Jana, saying there will be another two-hour wait. I still have 'low platelets', am still not much cop at keeping blood in so, she tells me, depending on what happens bleeding-wise 'on the table', that will determine whether she can do everything she wants to do today with the ... tissue scrape. Aaiieeee!

She tells me, for the first time, that what's happened to me is common, it's a 40 to 50 per cent fail-rate for all post-mastectomy reconstructions because of all the variables with individuals and chemo and radiation. 'It's not anyone's fault,' she reassures (I know she has to, in these outrageously litigious times), her warm brown eyes steady over her mask, today in full surgical blue scrubs, with a little hairnet. She reminds me about the possibility of the flap reconstruction in the future, if I want it. With a 40 to 50 per cent fail rate I doubt, now, I'll have anything glued to the front of my body ever again.

To pass the two-hour wait I read newspapers on my phone. There's an interview with William Shatner, sometime dreamy Captain Kirk, today something of a comedy maverick. He's asked what he knows at ninety that he wishes he'd known at twenty. 'Take it easy,' he advises, 'nothing matters in the end.' He adds, 'But if I'd known that at twenty, I wouldn't have done anything!'[2]

It's been a five-hour wait in total when a young nurse escorts me to the surgical ward, via the lift, where I see my reflection from every angle in the mirrored interior walls. I double-take, stunned. I look so frail, significantly more so than ninety-year-old Shatner, seemingly four feet tall, cheeks caved in, wearing a grandma's hospital hairnet, woolly grey slippers on the end of orthopaedic socks and the billowing hospital nightie.

What the hell has happened to me!?

In the anaesthetic room just outside the theatre, a friendly anaesthetist explains everything she's doing, gives me an oxygen mask and I drift off, into oblivion, unlike being electrocuted on the operating table back in the so-called swanky, private hospital.

Waking up in the recovery room there's now a huge, honeycomb-style dressing where The Monster once was. After obs, a cup of tea and a finger of shortbread, I'm wheelchaired back to the original ward for another two-hour wait. The surgeon visits again, says everything went well and she was able to scrape as much as she'd hoped. Groooo!

Wheelchaired out of the hospital, Ev is there in the car park once more and I'm inching towards her with a blood drainage bottle once more, which I was not expecting, a tube inserted into my side with its own square dressing. This being an NHS hospital, they don't do fetching polka-dot Drain Dollies. Instead, my bottle of blood is tipping over at 45 degrees in a Sainsbury's plastic bag.

Back at home, the pain feels as bad as it did after the actual mastectomy. For a few days I take codeine as sparingly as I can, eye twitching towards the box of laxatives, and watch more episodes of *The Repair Shop*. The mouth ulcers flare up again, the pain from the tube wedged inside my body so sharp I'm shuffling around the flat like Old Man Steptoe. I'm also back to the showerless life, dumped in the paltry puddle bath.

The drainage tube is scheduled for removal in the breast clinic, which necessitates a Covid test at the hospital the day before. I walk to and from both appointments, four long hours each day, plodding my way like the bent-over silhouettes in the road traffic warning signs: 'Caution! Old folk crossing!'

On the journey there Ali rings and I tell her I'm doing a reccy on the way home of hairdressers to see if there's anything they can do to resurrect the patchwork sadness of my damaged hair without the use of bleach, which would make the lot fall out, the follicles still too fragile.

'But I'll be looking for deals because the robbers down here charge a hundred and thirty quid.'

'That's outrageous!' she roars, 'I get mine done for fifty.'

It's the first time I've visited a proper salon for years, financially constrained to a cheapo, one-bleach-fits-all option. There are no deals in any of the local hairdressers. It's early summer and as expected, I'm quoted £130 for a half-head of namby-pamby, bleach-free highlights, cut-and-blow-dry, which I know I can't afford. Worse, I'm advised to wait two more months until the Rod Stewart tuftiness has further grown in. Arriving back at the flat, dejected, Simon is home from his daily walk, counting out twenty-pound notes.

'Been turning tricks in the park, have we?'

'It's from Ali,' he says. 'She's just transferred it to my account, for you. For your hair.'

I ring Ali up to thank her and sob like a six-year-old child.

I'm lying yet again on a hospital day bed, as the breast nurse tugs painfully at the tube still dangling out of my body. It's stuck, it must be manoeuvred around, to loosen up. Suddenly ... it's out! The relief is instant, the week-long throb of pain simply turned off like a tap. The large surgical dressing over the site of the reconstruction is yet to be removed and I know I'll be heavily scarred underneath, but this is the most normal I've felt for months: The Monster is gone, this is my real body and there's finally no pain.

Two days later I see my one-breasted self in the living-room mirror for the very first time. And gasp out loud.

Oh no.

I'm staring at a mangled torso. It looks like I've been in a car crash involving burns, the radiotherapy having turned my chest wall a mottled, burnished brown. It's as if a large patch of elephant's hide has been grafted onto my body, horizontally split in two by a row of stitches, then sliced down the middle with another row of stitches, the top section folding into the bottom section, creating ridges and undulating puckers. It also looks like mountainous terrain, as seen from space. Or the face of a very angry, eyeless cat. It's so much worse than I ever thought it could be.

Days later a breast nurse hands me my new bosom in a plastic medical bag, a triangular, soft beige pouch full of what appears to be pillow stuffing. I smile wryly, thinking the last time I stuffed my bra I was ten years old, with Ali, arranging socks inside my big sister's bras pretending we were fully grown women, because fully grown women were something to do with bosoms, though we weren't quite sure why, not yet.

After weeks with the beige pouch, I'm fitted with a more robust option, a state-of-the-art prosthetic 'breast form'. Sitting in a spa-like environment inside the Northern which I did not know existed, a busy nurse opens and closes a dozen drawers in a wall of drawers, searching for just-the-right-fit of said form, in size and consistency. She's also fitting me with a bra, which has pockets either side, into which you slide the prosthesis, two hundred pounds-worth of silicone doing its very best to resemble a disembodied breast, in both look and feel, the most advanced available on Earth. (Before the 1970s, when silicone arrived, they were made of highly pungent rubber, pouches filled with tiny glass beads or inflatable prosthetics known to be problematic on flights, where pressure changes in the cabin caused involuntary expansion and occasional outright explosion.) I'll now have this for many years, until it breaks, or I choose to buy a different one, the NHS no longer funding, quite rightly, either my bras or my single, pretend bosom.

Knockers. I contemplate again my lifelong lack of fixation and can't recall, even once, having The Cleavage on display. Apart from that day in Jamaica when Shaun Ryder announced, 'You've got massive tits, man!' – although I was in a rock stars' swimming pool alongside him at the time. I've had them groped a few times by strangers while fully clothed in public (both men and women), didn't bother wearing a bra for a few years in the nineties (I suspect The Revolution was involved) but they've been particularly appreciated by Simon, a child of the 1970s whose first crushes were bosomy dollybirds off the telly.

I remember being transfixed by the sight of Mariah Carey's magnificently buoyant bosoms in 2005, crashing together, braless, under a tight, white, sleeveless T-shirt, like a pair of bouncing new-born caramel labradors as she relaxed on an undulating massage chair in her mansion in the Hollywood Hills. I've seen and felt the primal, sexual attraction, even as a heterosexual woman, for a lifetime. But they've never been a focus, for me, of my own body, never defined any notion of womanliness, even if they definitely work for sexual pleasure just like everyone else's.

But my sexual self has been suspended for so long I barely connect them to sex any more. I'm still not ready to return. I know I must be in denial, but at least I *do* know I'm in denial. I turn my back to Simon when I take my clothes off, to put night clothes on. Often, he'll reach over and stroke my back, letting me know he sees me, and still wants to touch me. The emotions are so conflicting I'm shutting them out, still: the horror at the mutilation, the gratitude for my life, the shame of not being 'there' for Simon (who swears he doesn't care). The truth is, since illness happened, since chemo robbed my libido, I'm just not that *bothered* about sex. I'm not that interested. I'm even beginning to think, in disbelief, I might have ... had enough?

I still think Simon is a very attractive man: when we first met I always used to think, when I opened my eyes in the morning and saw his enormous, pale blue eyes, raven's wings eyebrows and tantalising 'Elvis' lips, it was like looking in a jewellers' shop window. 'Look at you,' I'd blurt out loud, 'hunkin' away!' If anything, he's even *more* attractive to me now, as a fifty-year-old man, the love I feel for him even deeper, perhaps because these last two years have fused us together so tightly, and tested us, and proved the strength of our bonds.

I think about sex sometimes, of course. I even bought a tasteful, lipstick-sized vibrator from that cradle of erotica, Sainsbury's, which I've had a go on, privately, to see if it reignited the low-flickering embers. It sort of did. But not by much. This is uncomfortably uncool, I know: women my age are bombarded daily by messages telling us our sexual selves are vital, without which we're barely alive. Newspapers and TV experts are forever on hand with how-to guides on reversing this disastrous development, insisting you must schedule 'maintenance shags' otherwise, the inference goes, it's your own fault if you're chucked, saucy interviews forever on *This Morning* with Iris, the eighty-something grandma about her ongoing 'steamy' jungle-sex with her thirty-something Egyptian husband Mohamed. Go for it, I say, to both of them. Me? If I was single now, I'd be more inclined to agree with Simon's eighty-four-year-old Aunty Joan in Wales, who once told me, when it came to sex, 'Oh, I can't be bothered with all that *nonsense* any more.' I see the Instagram photos of Madonna, her new alien head thrust under the bed out of sight, splayed legs in fishnets inviting the world to stare at her butthole and I think, Seriously? Is this *all* you are now?

Sometimes, when myself and Simon are in bed together and hooting like kids at some silliness, I think this is more meaningful, intimate and pleasurable to me now than sex ever was anyway. At least, that's how I feel for now. Things may change. (Maybe I've just forgotten ...)

It will be months before I can bring myself to show Simon the wreckage of my torso. And when I do, he is gentle, of course.

'I thought it would be worse,' he says.

And yes, by then, it's *been* worse. But it will always be very ugly. And I'll live with it. Because the word 'live' exists in that sentence and that is all I need. And when he wraps me in his arms in bed every single night, I know he can feel, on the right side, that there's nothing there. But *I'm* there. And today we're still too relieved about that to feel sad about anything else.

31

THIS COULD BE THE LAST TIME

On the early morning walk to chemotherapy for the very last time, in summer 2021, I remember the changing of the seasons these last eighteen months on these very same streets: boots crunching into gravel-strewn ice or splatting through rain, the curiously thrilling crinkle of freshly fallen leaves, the PVC of some much-admired comedy ankle boots melting as if candlewax in the Italy-level sunshine of summer 2020.

More than any of that, though, I remember the sound of the first lockdown, the birdsong tweeting in the treetops, birdsong which had always been there but no one heard, obliterated by the delivery vans, school-run saloons and worker-ferrying buses. Today, that birdsong, once again, is undetectable. Those loud, merry, new-day chirrups are lost, once more, in the scoosh and rumble of permanent London traffic. Has anything, I wonder, in this summer of wildfires torching the planet and metropolis subway floods, really changed?

After eighteen months of chemotherapy, surgery, radiotherapy, more surgery and more chemotherapy, I'm sitting in a reclining chair watching my NHS dream team care for what they're now calling 'newbies', patients at the beginning of their scenic expedition to the very edges of themselves. Prince puts his arm around me and I burst out blubbing. A faint, familiar swell of strings tinkles out from the radio on reception.

It can't be, can it? You're havin' a laugh!

They're playing 'Wind Beneath My Wings'. Tears trickle once more but this time I'm smiling, remembering the rain-lashed car journey with Ali to Stonehaven in late 2019, when I was convinced I was about to die. They're now tears of relief and gratitude – and an inner mirth that this, of all songs, is playing now, of all times.

Nadia hoists my chemo drip bag onto the pole with the castors and I hand her a gift for the unit: a card with a wonky rainbow illustration and a box of swish Belgian biscuits, like the ones I used to look forward to so much in the early, miserable months. She takes the package to reception, and I hear her and Prince laughing.

To ... Nadia, Bimpe, Prince, Kevin, Mel, Linda, Sheila, Sandie and everyone else who's taken care of me in the ever-moving chemo suite since January 2020.

The words 'thank you' can never be enough for everything you've done for me over the last eighteen months ... i.e. doing everything you can to save my life! The NHS is this country's greatest achievement, and you are the very best of us ... it's absolutely true. I salute you all, for your expertise, kindness, gentle hands, humanity, integrity and good humour ... and all through a global pandemic (absolutely none of which applies to the recently resigned health secretary!*).

Your dedication to your work and every one

---

*Matt Hancock, from several political lifetimes ago, whose 'job' eighteen months from now is chomping on camel penis for applause in the Celebrity Jungle.

of your patients has been awe-inspiring to witness and all I can do is say thank you and give you some biscuits. As well as all my gratitude for ever.

All the very best to you all ...

Sylvia (the Scottish one with the excellent port!) xxxx

Nadia returns, eyes sparkling above her mask, saying 'I love the card, "The Scottish one with the port!"' Me, I cannot speak. On the radio they're now playing Take That's 'Back For Good', which makes me both choke and simultaneously smile. Am I back? For good? I have a mammogram due on the remaining, oven-glove breast in two weeks' time, and that's when I'll truly know.

An hour later Nadia takes the needle out of my excellent port for the very last time. I'm staring at her in wonder, knowing she's as efficient and kind with everyone else, every day of her working life.

'You'll just carry on now, won't you, Nadia?'

'We'll be busy from tomorrow, very busy, more and more patients, because of the Covid backlog ...'

'You just ... do it, don't you!'

'Yes! We just do it.'

I slide off the chair and head out from behind the blue curtain to say goodbye to all the others, a lump forming in my throat, not knowing how I can possibly thank them enough in person.

'They're in a meeting!' hoots Nadia.

Oh. Of course they're in a meeting, these people are very busy! Much too busy to be listening to the likes of me weeping and thanking and fumbling. She escorts me through the door and I thank her all over again even if I know, by now, she should be *throwing* me out of the suite.

'Take care, Nadia!'

'Thank you ... and we will keep the card!'

I blub all the way along the corridor, into a lift, down the stairs and out the front door, knowing I'll never see these people again. Well, apart from two more bone infusion treatments over the next twelve months. Or if, of course, I'm diagnosed with this particular disease all over again in the future. But who knows what the future holds for any of us?

It's a curious fact of prolonged hospital treatment – when you continually see the same nurses, doctors and surgeons – how anonymous you must remain. There's simply no time for 'getting to know you' pleasantries; you're just one individual among a revolving door of infinite individuals, over many punishingly busy years. You're first and foremost a malfunctioning machine and the NHS staff are the engineers and mechanics there to fix your broken crankshaft, and all the rest of it, as fast and efficiently as they possibly can. To this end, all the NHS staff need to know is your age, whether you're allergic to anything, any important medical history, what's wrong with you and what they're doing to try to fix you. Everything else is irrelevant: your country of birth, background, job, class, salary, ethnicity, sexuality, gender, lifetime achievements, lifetime tragedies, everything which constitutes your personal sense of identity. Which is why, one day – on a routine, face-to-face check-up – it's so disconcerting when the wall of anonymity suddenly detonates.

'I saw you on TV!' blurts Keren the breast nurse, a huge smile on her face.

It's March 2021 and I'm sitting on the edge of the consultation bed, legs dangling, preparing to take my shirt and bra off so they can inspect the flaming red octopus head stuck to my body, days after the BBC repeated the 2018 documentary *Top of the Pops: The Story of 1986*, where I'd briefly appeared going on about my beloved Housemartins, the comedy Marxist, agit-pop heroes and self-anointed 'fourth best band in Hull'. I'm rumbled; they now know that I was, and occasionally still am, a music journalist.

'We didn't know you were a celebrity!' exclaims the powerhouse consultant surgeon Ms Mariam Jana, the trio ignoring my corrective protestations and bursting with questions instead, over the magazines I've worked for and which of the fabulous famous I've met, with unexpected queries arriving from Greek-born Martha as to the precarious condition of sauce-crocked, Celtic-punk bum Shane McGowan. Three faces beam at me with palpably delighted eyes, as I internally cringe with the lunacy of their sudden new perception. We all know, and I know *they* know, it is they who are the impressive ones, who prolong and actually save lives, and yet, for some minutes, I'm more interesting to them than they are to me, or even to themselves. It's testament to the power of illusory fame, and a reminder to me, at a time when showbiz had retreated to the furthest backburner of my life, of how we're all, to some degree, suckers in the court of the famous, forever curious over the hidden world of The Stars. Sometimes, it's merely the surface thrill of amusing or scandalous gossip, sometimes acknowledgement of the heroes of our adolescence and beyond, and all of it, ultimately, is testament to the human need for culture, a civilising force, as much as fire, sanitation and empathy. I sense a welcome light relief for them, too, in their none-more-important and often harrowing daily work.

Soon, though, the specks of stardust dissipate, as they always do, and reality returns, as it always does, and I'm once again just one more malfunctioning machine, my disfigured bare torso exposed to the ceiling, looking for answers to my individual problem which only they can provide. They are experts in their field who won't look back, as we patients do, on what they did for us, only forward onto the next patient, while we fade from view and become, at best, I like to think, 'the cheery Scottish one with the interesting shoes' (even when I didn't feel particularly cheery).

In summer 2021, post-implant removal operation, I have my final appointment with the surgeons, about which I feel embarrassingly sentimental. In familiar corridors I wait outside their consultation room and try not to fret over the words I need to conjure to thank them sufficiently for everything they've done for me. The door opens and a stranger's head appears, a young nurse I don't know, 'The doctor is ready for you.'

The doctor? *Surgeons aren't called doctors . . .*

Walking in, I'm staring at a second stranger, who says, 'Hello, I'm one of the consultants,' and I recognise his voice. He phoned the other week to see how I was as Ms Jana and Martha were busy. He remembers I had a concern: a stray stitch has been left in a wound, while around the surgical area remain surges of pain and a burnished chest wall still worryingly hard to the touch. Lying face up on the couch, right arm behind my head, exposing the ruched elephant's hide to two complete strangers, I'm dismayed that they're not My Team. Where are my women? Where are *my* surgery pals!?

The perfectly reasonable doctor observes the stitch, snaps on blue surgical gloves, removes a steel scalpel and hook from its packaging, and begins to pull, gently, at the stitch, until he has to pull more rigorously (without anaesthetic) . . . and it's out. It's dangling on the hook, gone. Again, instantaneous relief. I ask about the soreness, about the hardness, about not being able to lie on my natural sleeping side, still. Only time, I'm told, will improve things. The nurse is pleased I mention Bio-Oil, which I'm now using at Ali's suggestion, to help with scars. 'It will all soften and become smooth and flat,' she assures, which seems unlikely to me now, but she will have seen It All.

'You can get dressed,' informs the doctor, 'and we'll see you next year.'

I'm stunned. Is that it? I won't see my surgery pals ever again? Maybe not. But let's *hope* not. Because I'll only see them again if there's something wrong with the mammogram on the breast that remains, a test scheduled for 15 July. I don't ask where my pals are because I know where they are; busy with other patients, busy being surgeons, busy in an operating theatre with women whose needs are significantly greater than mine right now and possibly ever were. I feel, though, momentarily bereft.

There'll be no more jokes about shoes. No more of Martha's head peering around a door exclaiming, 'There you are, beautiful!' (Even though I've heard her say this to everyone.) The last time Ms Jana rang for a routine check-up she'd said to me, 'You've cheered us up! And you've been very strong.' The thought of those words makes me weep, openly, as I walk down the corridor from her consultation room for the very last time, these warm, encouraging words from a woman who had seen me at my most vulnerable, inferring I had somehow helped *them*. I remember the last time I saw her in person, on a post-implant removal check-up, when she'd complimented my black-and-white chequered mask.

'Look, today even your mask matches your shirt!' she'd exclaimed, and it did.

'Standards!' I'd quipped, as my elephant's hide creaked below my swirly black-and-white shirt, 'you've got to attempt *some* standards.'

So, there had been no proper goodbye with them, either. But who needs that in their situation anyway? A procession of healed patients lunging around their shoulders (especially in Covid times), declaring them angels and heroes, while another woman currently white-knuckled on a plastic chair ten feet away could be moments from being told, by them, she has incurable, metastatic stage four breast cancer and one year to live. They care, of course they care, they're all about The Care, but we are, ultimately, just fleetingly observed, broken-down machines. We will never really know each other because we don't have to, because that was never the point. The point is, and it's worth saying over and over again, that we who live in these often-beleaguered isles have access to, 'from cradle to grave', our NHS, for free, which isn't just a privilege – it makes us among the most fortunate human beings who have ever lived.

32

IT AIN'T OVER 'TIL IT'S OVER

July 2021.

I'm back at the mammogram machine, my remaining, oven-glove breast gripped inside the vice, my last hospital appointment for the foreseeable future. Twenty months on from the first mammogram and the circle is complete. I've been having a thorough feel at home for months, nothing has been detectable.

Doc Bridger has said, 'I'm not expecting anything,' and with all that zappery over eighteen months there can't be a single dodgy cell left. Surely? I don't feel nervous or frightened but nonetheless I'm scrutinising the face of the radiologist sitting silently at her screen, locking onto her eyes above her mask, for any sign, any twitch, any acknowledgement that there's something there, something that might cause her to say, 'It's a lot to take in.' Because if there is, I'll have to do what I've just done, for another eighteen months, *all over again*. Not a quiver of an eyelash detected.

I head out towards the tube, myself and Simon now off on our first actual holiday since 2019, two nights in dreamy Cambridge, our treat for making it through the 'best' part of two years of daunting, painful and double-isolated personal and global madness. The Covid vaccines have worked. The planet is waking up.

It's a stunning, sun-baked summer's day and we're sitting

with our bare feet in the river Cam, having just been goosed by, er, an angry swan, my arms stretched outwards, overcome with a feeling of intense freedom. And, yes, happiness. As much happiness as I've ever known. Even if I am currently mutilated, unemployed, have zero future security and a kitchen that's been falling apart for years. For now, I have everything I could possibly need: Simon, my friends and family, a blue sky, the river which runs through a beautiful, historical town, two bottles of rosé wine in a plastic bag full of ice cubes and a body that isn't trying to kill me any more.

Unless, of course, *it still is*?

2 August 2021, 9.50 a.m.

'Hello, this is Dr Bridger here, I'm early for once!'

All the liquid inside my mouth immediately dries up as my heart begins thumping beneath my ribs.

Oh God, she's never early, she's always late . . . it must be urgent . . . I'm doomed!

'. . . I'm calling with your mammogram results and they're fine, nothing to worry about.'

'Really? Completely fine!?'

'They're fine, yes.'

In my head I'm thinking, *Fine?* Is that all? Not 'brilliant' or 'the most cancer-free breast tissue in history'? But 'fine' I will take.

'So do you have the appointment for your bone infusion?'

'Yes, December!'

'Good. And I've booked you in for a heart scan in November, which I'm sure will be fine . . . and you're still taking the Letrozole?'

'Yes.'

'Good. And you'll have an annual mammogram now for four years . . .'

'OK. And then . . . well . . . is that it, then?'

'It is, yes. Are you starting to feel recovered now?'

'Oh, yes. Almost normal. Ish!'

'And your mouth is OK?'

'All good!'

'Great. Well ... I think you should go on holiday!'

'Well, I wish I could say the same to you, but I bet you're not going on holiday! And thank you so much for everything you've done – not only for me, but all the other hundreds if not thousands of women in your care, you are absolutely fantastic at your job.'

'Oh! Well, thank you very much ... but I'll speak to you after your heart scan in November. Are there any other questions for me?'

'Just the chemo port really, which is still there ...'

'Ah, of course! I'll request a date for removal.'

'Great. So ... until November ... take care.'

'And you. Bye!'

The fabulous 'Dr Badger' disappears, an exceptionally efficient professional who will no doubt have, like the surgeons, significantly less good news to impart to others on this sunny late-summer's day. But in my case, and in countless more cases like me, this particular doctor and the NHS she works for have unquestionably saved my life. Again. Simon's been standing feet away listening and we both brim with tears, waves of relief washing over us like the cool, calming waters of the river Cam over our feet only one week ago. *We made it.*

Ali rings asking how Cambridge was and I'm suddenly aware of a change in my voice; it's so much stronger. There's been a faint husk detectable for eighteen months which I'd stopped noticing. Now, I hear clarity, as the ravaged throat heals itself on the miraculous cellular level, now that my immune system exists once more. I'm also talking more than her, for once, with a detectable inner buoyancy. I sound ... normal. In fact, better than normal, more alive than normal, *back from the dead* normal. Like a cryogenically frozen human being, perhaps, brought out of the liquid nitrogen storage tank and laid out in the upcoming sunrise, thawing out, senses reigniting, astonished, ecstatic at being given another chance.

My hopeless hair, meanwhile, is also in urgent need of being brought back to life. By September, I'm striding into the swish Muswell Hill salon where I'd found the most sympathetic advice that summer, clutching an envelope with Ali's hundred pounds, an additional twenty-five pounds from Simon's mum for my birthday back in March, which I'd kept specifically for this event, and ten pounds of my own to cover the bill and a five-pound tip (c'mon, £130 for a standard hairdo is scandalous enough as it is). Two hours and six inches of hair on the floor later, expert male Italian hands are flicking at a bouncing, short-ish bouffant, while his eighteen-year-old apprentice coos around me. 'Oh, that's lovely! So much better!' (Which wasn't difficult.) The highlights are non-bleached, subtle but effective, the limp, mousy-brown sadness now a dancing, golden shimmer. Because of the thin, weedy condition, and still growing-in sides, the normally one-length affair now has perky layers, short at the front, which my Italian friend has whisked upwards into undulating waves. This isn't my hair, it's a middle-aged, middle-class woman's hair. Even if I'm now counting out the cash from the white envelope onto the counter (with extra on my card seeing as I'm suddenly being charged £170, because this is London, innit?) like a daffy ninety-four-year-old counting out her pension in Muswell Hill's swankiest *salon de coiffure*.

Darting into a nearby pub loo to wet the hair, I stick my head upside-down under the dryer, shake out the weedy waves and let it lie wherever it wants to, like I always do. That's better. *Now* I have a new hairdo! And now I can see the difference a decent hairdo makes. It's not only my hair that's lighter, it's me. It seems to have changed my skin, which is ... *brighter*. I don't look like a sick person any more. I look *almost* like I used to. When I was living the miracle of normality.

In the following weeks, there will be a further reignition, the return of the dormant libido. After almost two years of a chemical, shock, and stress-induced flatline, that, too, is waking up. There are tentative moves at first, but we're getting bolder, getting over the self-consciousness, getting used to the new normal. But the flame, still, for me physically, remains abnormally low. It's only now, though, that I google possible side effects for Letrozole, that 'oestrogen-blocking treatment' so bewilderingly noted on The Doc's original treatment plan a lifetime ago, tablets I now take every day and must take for a full five years. It's an 'aromatase inhibitor, which can reduce sexual desire'. So, while things may not be what they were, perhaps there's a winking light on the horizon: the sixty-one-year-old me, finally off the pills, even *worse* (i.e. better) than steamy Iris, the perky eighty-something grandma.

For we survivors, at least I now know, it's all just part of 'the process'.

33

ANY PORT IN A STORM

The port which has saved me from striking veins for eighteen months is being removed today, in late September 2021. It's a seemingly straightforward procedure happening in the day-care centre where the chemo ward was moved to in late spring 2020, when the world was first broken by Covid.

Walking through the familiar front doors I remember how feeble I was back then, how painful, miserable and debilitating everything was, how long the road ahead felt. I remember, too, the visible panic of the bustling technicians, hastily reconfiguring a surgical recovery room into a suite full of digital pump machines, reclining chairs and cold cap refrigerators. It's astonishing, I marvel, how resilient the NHS has been. And how positively Amazonian, compared to then, I now feel. Which is to say *inches* away from normal, other than a tenderness inside the cheeks, which now feel permanently scarred. But there's no pain. No pain! And that's all I'll ever need.

Once again, I'm lying on an operating table, but this time wide awake. The room is busy, surgical assistants everywhere, maybe six. One of them says, 'Are you cold? Are you all right? Don't look so frightened!' I'm not aware I'm frightened, but the eyes, wide over the mask, must betray me. It's not every day, after all, you invite someone to wield a scalpel at your neck.

The port is situated just under the right collarbone, which attaches, via catheter tube, to a major vein in my neck. The surgeon arrives and introduces himself, a Greek man called Andrew, with soft, calm brown eyes above his mask. A blue surgical fabric suddenly flaps overhead and descends around my ears, landing flush onto my face. 'It's on her face!' shouts a nurse, as hands shoot under the blue to lift it off and upwards, forming a tent which now surrounds my head and upper body. I'm told I can lower my mask now, a hand reaching into the tent to lower it for me. Andrew now says those familiar words, 'Sharp scratch,' as he begins the local anaesthetic injections, which penetrate deep into the flesh around both my collarbone and lower neck like brutal dental injections, my eyes watering, body tensing up. This is suddenly very real.

'Would you like some music?' someone asks. Not really, I'm thinking, I'm not in a spa here awaiting a massage, but if they insist ...

'Er ... some classical?'

Someone fiddles with a smartphone and music blares into the room, the demonic choir, apocalyptic tuba, portentous timpani and threatening strings of *Carmina Burana*, which only ever conjures associated thoughts of seventies' horror film *The Omen*, the word 'Damien' and horrific death. Help!

'Maybe a bit too dramatic!' I squeak, under the tent.

Andrew asks, 'Who's your favourite composer?'

'Beethoven,' I tell him and now the beautiful and funereal 'Moonlight Sonata' begins weeping into the room.

'Er ... maybe a bit sad!?'

The last time I heard this music, over and over again, was via Glasvegas, my last full-blown new-band-crush, who's street-gang opus 'Stabbed', released in 2008, was a spoken-word plea set to 'Moonlight Sonata' with the opening lyrics, in the purest Glaswegian accent, *I'm gonny get stabbed ...'*

'How about some eighties' music?' asks someone, helpfully, who's evidently taken in my age, and suggests, 'George Michael?'

'George is good!' I squawk, attempting to loosen up my body, which is now as rigid as rigor mortis, thinking as long as it's not 'Wake Me Up Before You Go-Go'.

'And I am Greek!' pipes Andrew, in a nod to his shared heritage with George Michael, as the sound of 'Careless Whisper' comes wafting, soothingly, into the room, followed by the sumptuously delicate 'Father Figure'. I begin, at last, to thaw.

'What's your job?' asks Andrew.

An inward chuckle. 'You'll never believe this ... a music journalist.'

'Oooh!' enthuse several voices, as a flurry of questions arrive. 'Who d'you work for? Who have you met?'

Suddenly, a penetrating stab, heading upwards, as if my collarbone is being gouged out.

'Uuuuuuh!' I say.

'More local,' instructs Andrew, 'more local ...'

My hands are now gripping the side of the surgery table, knuckles white. I can feel the scalpel deep inside my throat and I'm shaking. I must stop shaking, there's a man with a blade at my throat! Who's trying to microscopically scrape something away from a main artery.

'It's hanging on,' he says.

So am I, mate: another quiver from me and I'm *doomed*.

The staff are now asking Andrew where he comes from in Greece and I wish, in all honesty, they were concentrating on the hole in my neck (even if they *are* concentrating, they just do this stuff every day).

A penetrating pain.

My voice squeaks out, strained and compressed. 'I can feel it!'

'More local, more local!' implores Andrew as anaesthetic implements are swiftly handed over. Now he wants to know who's the best pop star I've ever met, the nicest, and I can't do this – 'I can't, I can't!' – not while there's a blade inside my throat and shouldn't I, you know, not really be talking seeing as talking is made from vibrations in the throat?!

I feel a tug-tug-tug, Andrew trying to free the catheter from the vein. It's stuck, I know it's stuck as much as the surgeon knows it's stuck.

'How long have you had the port?' he wonders.

'Eighteen months.'

Silence from everyone, finally.

I know a bit about this stuff – because of the Mechanical Chest and the capsular contracture catastrophe – about how tissue grows around foreign bodies. Eighteen months of tissue growth around a tube, I'm now imagining, will be like fibreglass insulation compacted in a wall.

He slices deeper. I feel it, the pain bone-deep and sharp.

'Ugh!'

'More local ... more local ...'

It now feels like I'm having my throat slit, my hands crushing the sides of the bed, as fingers now edge onto my fingers, a nurse, somewhere beyond the blue head-tent. She's willing me to grip onto her instead, which I do, and it's a small hand, and I might be hurting her, but I can't release this desperate grip, as the tug-tug-tugging carries on. This human touch makes me weep, tears seeping out from the sides of mascaraed eyes (eyelashes by now fully grown back). Talk starts up again, about living in north London, which I can't join in with, even as questions are asked – 'Hnn! Sorry!' – as the tug-tug-tugging suddenly ... stops.

'It's out.'

'Whoooo.'

A cold flannel appears in the tent, a nurse presses it onto my glistening forehead and dabs away the black streaks heading towards my ears. Stitches are sewn, a pressure dressing affixed and my grip loosens on the bloodless fingers of the surgical assistant, who gently pulls them away.

The tent comes off.

'Thank you!' I blurt to the assembled and see the assistant whose fingers I've crushed. 'And thank you so much for your hand, even if you made me cry!'

She merely smiles, as Andrew tells me everything went well, no problems at all. He advises I don't do any swimming for a while, making expansive swimming gestures. I promise him I won't be swimming – I'll be sitting down, possibly in a pub, soon. His dark-brown eyes twinkle, full of warmth and confidence and skill and empathy. He winks and disappears from the room.

Wheeled into a recovery room, there's a woman in the bed opposite, moaning and sobbing, the blue curtain soon swinging around her for privacy. For two hours I'm staring at the '3 a.m. Eternal' ceiling tiles, listening to the chat between nurses, about Covid and holidays cancelled and the lack of a proper pay rise. Andrew reappears to check I'm still OK. I'm definitely still OK.

'Take care,' he says, with a friendly and very gentle punch to my arm. This is what the NHS can do, then, on its knees, still in the midst of a global pandemic, in autumn 2021.

And now I'm becoming more fixed by the day, thoughts turn to something else that desperately needs fixing: Sad Kitchen.

34

YOU'LL ALWAYS FIND ME IN THE KITCHEN AT PARTIES

In summer 2021 I look afresh at my coffers with the windfall and think: Maybe, now, I can add to that. Because of Covid I've spent very little for a second year. Simon, too, in these non-spendy times, can make a sizeable contribution. I've also kept money aside for my funeral for years (the inner goth made me do it) and now, seeing as I haven't died after all, what am I waiting for, exactly? If both Covid and cancer have taught me anything it's to *get busy livin'*. To seize the day. The rainy day is now. Its name is Sad Kitchen.

When myself and Simon first started 'going out' in 2002, we spent weeks at a time talking about music – in pubs, living rooms, even bedrooms, on and on about this song and that lyric, cackling over the legendary quips from the musical renegades across our obsessive decades. Today, we're talking about *kitchens* for weeks – on and on about unit colours and worktops and induction cooker hobs which I've only ever seen on TV and can't believe are in any way affordable. It's mostly *me*, mind, who's going on and on – 'I don't care about colour coordination!' he scoffs, where I definitely *do* – and am therefore appointed Project Manager, despite making a shambles of it the first time, what with the useless romanticism, van Gogh fixation and zero common sense.

While I'm googling what it means to buy a kitchen (from where, who fits it and how much *does* it all cost anyway?), Simon confronts the miserable, water-damaged, tinfoil-blanketed window. We've found the source of the leak, which is more than the council ever has: a build-up of moss grown from pigeon shit clogging up the drainage gutters. Through creative ingenuity, a bottle brush attached to a wooden pole, courageous manoeuvres leaning out the window and what Simon calls his lengthy 'monkey arms', the rooftop pipes – finally! – are cleared. Within days, Sad Window in Sad Kitchen is a newly papered, painted, sanded and varnished window surround and window seat any estate agent would fanfare as A Delightful Period Feature. Now, we call the professionals.

Three comedy cockney geezers are singing their heads off to Absolute Radio, a constant croon of ye olde hit singles, from Dire Straits' 'Sultans of Swing' to Madness' 'It Must Be Love' to The Zutons' 'Valerie'. It takes them six swift days of singing, drilling, hammering, wiring, tiling and a bit more singing to create the actual Kitchen Of Our Dreams. Sad Kitchen has been cremated, Joyous Kitchen risen like a wooden, steel and ceramic phoenix from spidery graveyard ashes.

We have wall cupboards. We've never had wall cupboards! The induction hob is science-fiction, a magnificent achievement in robotic technology and it 'talks' to you, bleeps when you switch it on, bleeps when you're turning it up or down, has a glowing red 'H' sign when the hob's still hot, wishing to keep you out of A&E. There's the hood above the hob – we've never had a *hood* – a stainless-steel chimney hoovering up all the upwardly coiling grease while the oven is 'pyrolytic' and can, therefore, clean itself via an inbuilt dirt incineration process (cor!).

The fridge/freezer also 'talks', bleeping when you've left the door open too long, while the washing machine works properly, doesn't need a pinging-off hose (and the old one never did: the original fitter, the plumber tells us, left a 'kink' in the plumbed-in hose). Everything works perfectly and everything is sparkling clean. The laminated wooden worktop will *never* turn to rot, all appliances are housed behind integrated, 'antique-white' shaker doors, no gaps, no grease and no crumbs creating archaeological strata ever again. Our new overhead light is a stunner, a large, matt-white pendant lamp, with a single bulb, its wide underside coated with high-glam copper which, when switched on, floods the newly painted white walls with a sumptuous, coppery glow. The new, refurbished Two Lamps is officially *open*.

One Saturday morning at 9 a.m., we're both sitting up in bed, phones aloft, googling and wondering out loud, 'What d'you think about *this?*' I'm ordering a new, *small* kitchen table, the day after the room-dominating Vincent has been carted off by the council. We also need new pots 'n' pans compatible with the induction hob and tempted by a no doubt huge sale lie I go for two-hundred pounds off a set of coppery Gotham Steel beauties befitting the likes of Nigella Lawson for ninety-seven pounds (a snip!).

Soon, I'm going mad. The new stainless-steel sink is so fabulously clean I can't bear the manky old washing-up bowl sticking up beyond the rim, so now I'm googling 'collapsible washing-up bowls', alongside 'under cupboard stick-on lights' for that all important Kitchen Disco experience. Simon is also fevered, ordering a small bamboo trolley with shelves and a new wooden chopping board because the old plastic one, too, is manky and we can't have *that* ruining our pristine Joyous Kitchen. So now we are the kind of people for whom the thrills of the Saturday morning sex-up have been comprehensively usurped by the joy of a copper-bottomed pan. Soon we will be OCD-level dirt police pouncing with brand new cloths should a crumb, flake or any blemish whatsoever appear on any surface, including *inside* the cupboards. I'm spending *hours* googling coordinated kettles and toasters, dish racks, placemats and coasters, while staring over at the gleaming, woody, white and ochre vision of one-wall sophistication.

'It's a grown-up's kitchen!' I yelp. 'I'm fifty-six and finally a grown-up!'

The self-assembly trolley arrives and within ten minutes Simon has built the top drawer.

'I've turned into a domestic man,' he beams, Allen key aloft. 'For the first time in my life I'm useful! Not like that typing fool for all these years.'

I can feel an inner smile bursting out of my body, an actual surge in the valves of my heart, for one specific reason: after these past two years of madness, after everything Simon's done for me, everything he's personally witnessed and tolerated, it was something I wanted to do for him, much more than for myself. And I did it. We did it. And he loves it. And he deserves it.

Here in London, barely a week goes by without local news footage of a broken human being, in a broken-down home, in tears, showing an appalled reporter around a damp, poisonous home, walls blackened with mould, buckets on floors collecting putrid water drip-drip-dripping through ceilings. If we ever wonder why homes matter so much, ask anyone whose home is a hovel. Money doesn't buy you happiness is the cliché's cliché, of course, but it certainly buys you options and freedom and the kind of pleasant domestic surroundings which form a perceived protection from the ugliness of much of reality. I know it's just a kitchen. I know none of this mattered when I thought I was about to die. I would happily have lived in an upturned wheelbarrow on a compost quarry in Clacton as long as I stayed alive. But now that I *am* staying alive, for a good while it seems, a gorgeous expanse of meticulously grouted ochre tiles beneath sturdy, pristine wall cupboards *doesn't half cheer you up*.

Clearing out the cluttered pantry one day I find a rarely opened box of household trinkets. There's an object inside I don't recognise, a round, two-part wooden gizmo that looks like both sides of a doorknob fitted together, the inside of the halves studded with small metal spikes. A jolt of memory, a gasp out loud.

'You're joking!'

It's a grinder for separating out your bushel of skunk weed, essential for the professional-level stoner I used to be through the rollicking 1990s. I haven't seen it for years, had forgotten I ever had it. I certainly don't need it any more. This ignites another memory: back in the summer of 1990, baseball-hatted DJ elf Adamski went to No. 1 with 'Killer', featuring enigmatic vocalist Seal. At the time, to me, it felt like The Revolution, a victory for the maverick outsiders, so I bought – for myself and flatmates Siân, Trish and Gilly B – a celebratory bottle of champagne. Today, thirty-one years later, a bottle of actual Bollinger sent by Jill from Abu Dhabi this summer, to toast the end of my chemo, still waits in the new fridge, bubbling with anticipation. We didn't get round to opening it, decided we'd wait until the kitchen was finished. That day is today.

Sipping the most expensive drink we've ever sipped in The Two Lamps by some distance, this is a very different kind of revolution. But a revolution all the same: a new-found respect for material surroundings, and why they matter so much, and why we should all take care of them, like I didn't, for far too many years. I think once more about my revolutionary teenage self, in ideological opposition to the stifling conventions of 'mortgages and fridges'. Today, I couldn't be more relieved to have a mortgage I can afford, and a towering integrated talking fridge.

Meanwhile, stowed away inside a quality wall cupboard is the old-school cake stand I bought from a charity shop in April 2021, so keen was I to fittingly commemorate the funeral of Prince Philip (as someone who'd always found Philip audaciously amusing). That nationally sombre day, I piled onto the florally decorated tiers a selection of crustless sandwiches and vanilla slices, raising a toast to Philip from the bottle of Captain Tom gin Ev had given me for Christmas. And that righteous revolutionary, the one who smoked marijuana on a clifftop in 'protest' at Charles and Diana's wedding, would've surveyed this scene in disbelief, convinced the real me had been abducted and replaced by a malfunctioning replicant grandma gone catastrophically soft in the head.

On this day, though – forty years on from that royal wedding, thirty-five years on from the release of The Smiths' *The Queen Is Dead* – and the monarchy is now, to me, a fascinatingly ludicrous cultural tradition and the most gripping soap opera on the telly, significantly less harmful to British society specifically and life on Earth generally than ceaseless crooks inside the Conservative government, fossil fuels, Big Tech, intensive global farming, internet disinformation and Vladimir Putin. Moreover, I still fully agree with my mum's regularly repeated refrain whenever ma'am appeared on TV: 'The Queen never put a foot wrong in her life.' Unlike most of the rest of them.

And the following year, 2022, when the Queen *did* die, in those compelling, bewildering, often beautiful days that followed, through all the arcane absurdism in ostrich feather hats – as the new Liz in town, Truss, readied herself for 'rule' (with immediate cataclysmic results) – the British monarchy seemed less and *less* like the most acutely pressing of our planetary problems.

If anything, it would be weirder if I *hadn't* changed in forty years, seen no shifting of perspective, priorities, or passions. Today, contemplating the home I'm privileged to own, I'm reminded of something Ev has said for years, Scottishly, as she's closed the front door on her own version of a sanctuary, safe from harm.

'Hame's best.'

35

THANK YOU FOR THE MUSIC

Alexa sits in the kitchen where it's been since Christmas 2019, now on the new, gratifyingly small table, causing me endless decision paralysis as to what I'd like to hear. All the music from The Olden Days, the music which formed me, including all that music I've written about with a fervour, at times, bordering on the psychotic, now often feels like over-chewed chestnuts decomposing on the floor of ancient woodlands. What we at *Smash Hits* used to call 'rock's rich tapestry' is now, to my ears, a faded, fraying magic carpet, no longer able to fly me to thrillingly different dimensions, as if its wizardly wings have fallen off in the handing down through the generations. I've been hearing the songs of my youth, now, for forty, even forty-five years, much of their power inevitably fading through the rusting properties of overfamiliarity. You can't take your old music, though, to *The Repair Shop*.

Occasionally, there'll be a kitchen disco chiefly powered by post-punk, flailing up and down the floorboards to the Neolithic hits of Adam And The Ants, Siouxsie And The Banshees, even bombastic, flint-faced goth ghouls Bauhaus, for a laugh. Mainly though, much more than my own teenage anthems, I turn to the even more venerable Greats, say, ver Stones, Neil Young and Joni Mitchell or the Small Faces, Sinatra and the Bee Gees in the sixties (before they became 'my' Bee Gees in the seventies). The eighties and nineties I rarely revisit: the Style Council soundtracked a spring clean once, there's a rare Oasis moment wondering if this music still 'works' (it does, only in the right mood ... oh man, it is LOUD), and if the mood is particularly buoyant a blast of the New Radicals 'You Get What You Give' from 1999 with its arms-aloft chorus *'You gotta reason to liiiiive!'*

Least often of all, though, I'll 'check out' the tunes of the young people, wonder if that new band everyone's going on about are actually any good or, as suspected, a weedy echo of The Fall. Findings: all right, I suppose, but a weedy echo of The Fall. And not as good as The Streets.

These habits tell the story. I still love music and listen to plenty, but I don't listen to the music of my youth, or to new music, the way I used to, any more.

It's been nothing to do with being ill, or believing I was about to die, and everything to do with advancing age, as it usually is for all of us. Unless, of course, it's still your job to seek out new music, or you're a fifty-something listener to BBC 6 Music, but even the 'cool' station of the middle-aged plays plenty of decades-old music (especially the only 6 Music shows I listen to, hosted by Iggy Pop and Huey Fun Lovin' Criminal).

In 2022 it's been forty-three years – *forty-three years* – since my personal musical year zero, 1979, aged fourteen, the year both glitterball disco and the post-punk insurrection forged my world view, igniting a passion for music not so much all-encompassing as my reason for living itself, which I turned not only into my work, but my lifestyle and pretty much my *life*.

Forty-three years before *that* it was 1936, the year the General Post Office introduced the speaking clock, the BBC's first public television broadcasts were beamed from Alexandra Palace, George Formby released 'When I'm Cleaning Windows', teenagers were still two decades away from being invented and Adolf Hitler was three years into his chancellorship of Germany with less than hilarious results.

Forty-three years in any aspect of culture is an epoch, it's archaeological *layers* of evolution and therefore every reason to have no idea whatsoever what the young people are on about, never mind listening to, watching, reading, or (more than anything) 'playing at' on their phones.

But it's not just ancients like me who aren't listening to young people's music any more; neither are the young people, at least not primarily, not in the way they used to pre-millennium. In 2018, comedy Glaswegian troubadour Lewis Capaldi, then twenty-two, told me he spent most of his tour downtime not listening to any music whatsoever but scrolling on his phone through comedy shows and podcasts, alongside *World War II In Colour*. 'I am a multi-faceted man!' he quipped, before adding his devotion to an Instagram page on dinosaurs. 'Dinosaurs are *class*.'

Teenagers today are as likely to be newly impassioned Beatles fans as were teenagers in the 1960s, or devotees of anything else from the past one hundred years, the history of popular music surrounding us twenty-four hours a day, every song ever released from every genre ever invented now as instantaneously accessed as electricity, and considerably cheaper (i.e predominantly free).

Here in London, perennial cradle of the youthquake, grime might be the dominant cultural force but in the high-street stores, charity shops, pubs (and, in my case, hospital wards), you're bombarded by The Olden Days, the classic hits of the twentieth century, from the fifties onwards, to the very early 2000s, at the latest, before digital life changed everything and the young were no longer purely products of their musical time. Streaming platforms are now dominated by the past, by what the industry calls 'catalogue' music by the ageing and the outright dead, artists in their late sixties, seventies and eighties commanding the biggest fiscal opportunities from selling off publishing rights (since 2019 alone, Bob Dylan, Paul Simon, Bruce Springsteen, Tina Turner, Neil Diamond, James Brown, David Bowie).

Bands don't split up and, if they do, they get back together again, clambering like middle-aged, born-again Bash Street Kids up the steps behind the stage of the nearest heritage festival, today's moist-eyed, youth-reliving wormholes for every old-school tribe and generation. But this isn't just about Classic Old Music and pining for The Greats; for Generation Nostalgia it's often any old music from their youth, whatever was there when *they* were there.

In autumn 2021, I interviewed bowler-hatted eighties' pop sap Debbie Gibson, then fifty-one, who was about to re-release her first two albums of perky teen-pop schmaltz, who'd spent years appearing on nostalgia tours in the States, most recently in 2019 with flame-haired eighties' 'rival' Tiffany and late eighties/early nineties boyband colossus New Kids on the Block.

'People are so hungry for everything nostalgic right now,' declared the charming 'Gibbers', who had new fans in their teens and twenties who weren't even there at the time but were 'obsessed' with all things eighties. Why did she think that was?

'Somewhere in the 2000s it was, "The eighties are back!"' she mused. 'And it's just never gone away. I think it's because, especially now, with what's going on in the world, people long to return to a simpler time. There was an innocence to that time and in terms of music, it was simple, hooky, melodic. I don't think everything great happened in the past and I don't want a time machine to take me back, I don't think a lot of people do. But they want that feeling. On the Mixtape tour with New Kids I saw people celebrating, I saw women especially bonding with their girls and I say "girls" because women are just grown-up girls! And they wanted to just reconnect with a time and a place that made them feel free.'

Where does this leave, though, the Young People's Music? Bombarding their TikTok feeds of course, the infinite tsunami of old music matched only by the incoming deluge of the new, every screen they're addicted to hosting the most increasingly crowded new musical source in history. No wonder, so often, they seek out The Greats instead. As a semi-employed music journo still on scores of PR mailing lists, press releases for new bands and artists blow daily into my inbox as if powered by the global jet streams at a faster rate than ever, young talents I will mostly never listen to because my time on Earth is running out. Because no matter how magical some of them are, and some of them surely will be, they won't shape me the way music once shaped me, because at this age I'm already *shaped*. No music can move you, ever again, the way music did in your myopically intense youth, the music that seared your identity, formed your world view, informed your politics, ignited your attitude and found you an alternative family. A metamorphosis that can only happen when you're working out who you are, which by definition means when you're young. And then it stays with you for ever. Because it's *in* you. It *is* you.

As a teenager, I once threw my radio at the wall, smashed it and broke it, because DJ Annie Nightingale had reminded me that fog-bound goth gonks Sisters of Mercy were playing in Edinburgh that night and I didn't have a ticket. I wouldn't do that, now, even if David Bowie came back from the dead and was playing Ally Pally five hundred yards away. The first year I joined *Smash Hits*, sporting a vertical eighties fright-wig and fluorescent green tights, I had a heated argument with some stinky indie boys who failed to see the merits of equally fright-wigged kitsch-punk heroes We've Got a Fuzzbox and We're Gonna Use It, becoming so furious I erupted into tears. That would not happen today with any amount of 'shade' thrown over the fabulous Wet Leg lady-force. (Today, I'm significantly more furious with a universe that snuffed out Jo Dunne from Fuzzbox at age forty-three, in 2012, six weeks after being diagnosed with cancer.) I've slept on pavements in unknown cities to see bands, hitchhiked down motorways in trucks with dubious dudes to see bands, slept in ditches at Glastonbury when my tent was stolen (and didn't even *see* the bands I'd come to see). I'm not doing that now, no matter how rousing the communal sing-along thrills of howay-the-lad Geordie Sam Fender.

I don't *need* new music the way I used to, for much more than a pleasant distraction, a singalong with pals, a kitchen disco or a window into the always intriguing psyche of a new generation, which ignites the occasional flare of new fandom (the arrival in 2019 of Billie Eilish, alongside the rest of the captivated planet). In 2022, I sat on the sofa wiggling along to Billie's headline Glastonbury set as thrilled as anyone there (I'd imagine), the TV shindig an annual highlight I never miss. But I'm never going back. I've done my time, 1986–2001. I know exactly what I'm missing. And what I'm not missing. And all who make the pilgrimage in the years and decades ahead will have just as much of a life-enhancing, humanity-loving, reality-escaping, synapse-shredding, hysteria-inducing, existentially joyous a caper as I definitely did for an abundance of unforgettable years. As I reach into the towering, talking fridge for an ice-cold can, on the way back from the sparkling toilet, past the bedroom with the bouncy mattress, under a roof, in the dry, unburnt and unlost. I guess I just don't need the chaos any more, either.

The language of the young, meanwhile, is not my language, exactly as it should be. They have their own values, passions and struggles, their own version of reality, their own technological terminology, all blockchains, metadata and already-entrenched NFTs (it'll always stand for the National Film Theatre to me, so pass the Werther's Originals, grandma).

Even artists' names are now an alien concept, as they should be, skewing the language to reflect the way they communicate, via the centrifugal force of their culture, The Phone: acronyms, abbreviations, all manner of colloquial slang, altered spelling, numbers, keyboard symbols and underscores (there's a band *called* underscores), names without capital letters, or all capital letters, the mysterious use of double vowels, or no vowels at all, or unpronounceable and made-up curiosities more befitting a Countdown conundrum. Barrelling into my inbox through early to mid-2022 alone were: Dvwn, SwitchOTR, CMAT, VLURE, Bdrmm, Amaarae, ayrtn, Dreamer Isioma, HAAi, keiyaA, Vegyn, BENEE, ekkstacy, BRKN LOVE, Ibeyi, RIVRS, ElyOtto, Nukuluk, niina, HVOB, Barkaa, BRIDEAR, Bas Jan, M(h)aol, msftz, mxmtoon, STAYC, glaive, 3REE, 100 gecs, Sycco, x/o, AR/CO, NoSo, SKAAR, p-rallel, ELLLL, BEMZ, M1llionz, Noya Rao, NLE Choppa, THE BLSSM, TOKiMONSTA, morgxn, RY X, XATIVA, Biig Piig, RYL0, JFDR, Chiiild, R U Init, SZA, DellaXOZ, Ashnikko, Luude, PHEM, Cassyette, H09909, CISI, Alissic, Yung Gwopp, Meduulla, EMBY, DATURA4, Bru-C, JAWNY, kwn, ODESZA, lozeak, Æ Mak, RIOPY, Alvvays, Powfu, SSGKobe, ctkrl, bb, Zzzahara, 5v, ZelooperZ, JAXN, the puntastic Dora Jar and the admirably havin'-a-laugh iamamiwhoami. And if you say that lot in quick succession it could well be what the internal cogs of Spotify's Discover Weekly algorithm actually sound like.

Must I care? Must I *need* to know? We only feel we do, surely, because of our old foe FOMO (yes, there's a band called FOMO). But that kind of FOMO has died in my heart for ever: the only thing I fear missing out on, now, is both a present and a future, a chance at ongoing life blissfully unconcerned with the latest bleeps from the metaverse.

There is one 'new' music which *has* been welcomed into my world. Via Simon, enabled by Alexa, the now dominant soundtrack to my life is, very unexpectedly, jazz. I'd spent decades loathing jazz, thought it meant the dissonant, melody-free squalls of the likes of Ornette Coleman, was unmoved by the weedy lilts of Ella Fitzgerald, refused to invite into an evening's merriment the horrors of Billie Holiday's 'Strange Fruit'. Now? Alexa bathes the coppery white walls in boogaloo swing and ecstatic trumpets, from the standard greats of Duke Ellington, Louis Armstrong and Django Reinhardt to musicians I'd never heard of – Bix Beiderbecke, Cannonball Adderley, Oliver Nelson. I've 'discovered' Miles Davis, who for decades I specifically loathed, or believed I loathed as a favourite of the pompous snobs. Until now he was the oft-repeated butt of a joke which originated from a chum in Scotland. 'Miles Davis?' he balked, as another chum blabbed on and *on* about his cassette collection of the trumpeting renegade, 'I'd rather listen to (moustachioed, bow-tied, seventies/ eighties TV presenter of *World of Sport*) Dickie Davis!'

The joys of listening to this music are manyfold: not only a voyage of musical discovery but a compelling lesson in the often-inhumane history of America, revolutionary sounds made by extreme characters in extreme circumstances, with mostly no lyrics, *all about the vibe*, in the formative jazz way. You can, therefore, have a conversation at the same time, as opposed to, say, leaping out of your seat and bawling every word of The Cult's 'She Sells Sanctuary' with your arms in a fist-pump frenzy. You find music you've never heard before, as the decades go on, when you're ready to. And other than jazz, when people ask me, as they still do, what I'm listening to these days, I tell them the truth: podcasts. And the distant sound of a woodpecker's drill in Ally Pally Park.

In 2019, before Covid shut down the music industry, I had a conversation with Primal Scream's Bobby Gillespie, the most evangelical, righteous rock'n'roll dream believer of his generation. We were in Tate Britain, viewing the harrowing war photographs of veteran British documentary photographer Don McCullen.

'Rock'n'roll is dead,' he announced, breezily. 'There's no counterculture any more, nobody flash any more. There's loads of records I like but there's no interesting characters, no Johnny Thunders, the music's a retread. It's shite! I'd much rather go to a talk by left-wing writers and philosophers than see bands. My kid said a few years ago, Christmas, granny was in the kitchen,

'Gimme Shelter' was on, she was singing along. He laughed and goes, "Dad, you can't expect me to like the music my granny likes," and I went, 'Totally!" My kids like grime, drill, that's where the edge is now, it's sexier, more violent, more glamorous.'

So wasn't he, too, at almost sixty years old, fading into history? Still in Primal Scream after thirty-five years, a touring band who've become, like every 'heritage' band, their own tribute act?

'No,' he insisted. "Cos it's my culture. So I'm allowed to do it.'

He looked around at the walls of the Tate, at this honouring of the venerable relics of cultural history.

'We're in an art gallery,' he opined. 'And there was expressionism, surrealism, all the movements and they had their time. And rock'n'roll's had its time. Rock'n'roll's just ... music for your granny!'

If my rock'n'roll generation is, then, a blip in time, I couldn't be more thrilled it was the one I lived in. Lucky stars, once again. The music which has soundtracked my life has been as vital to me as oxygen, this uniquely potent, primeval forcefield which not only saved me in adolescence but gave me my adult life. So I say thank you for the music. The songs I'm singing. Thanks for all the joy they're bringing. But now my ark is full.

And my ark has sailed.

36

PICTURE THIS

March 2022 and I'm back in Scotland for the first time in almost three years, today in Broughty Ferry, just outside Dundee. This is the riverside town where my big sister Liz has lived since 1981, a secondary-school teacher bringing up her family with her husband, now a mind-blowing seventy years of age. I'm visiting her at home with middle sister Jackie, who's bursting with excitement, not only because it's the first time we sisters have been together for seven years, but because Liz has a surprise. She's looked out a large brown suitcase of old family photos, a cache we did not know existed, decades upon decades, stretching back to our Victorian grandparents, diligently collated selections gathered in plastic A4 pockets and individually titled: 'Mum', 'Dad', 'Billy', 'Ronnie', 'Liz', 'Jackie', 'Sylvia'. She also has all the documentation from my father's years in the Second World War, which Jackie originally sourced and gave to her for safekeeping. But I've never seen these treasures before. I pick up his 'Soldier's Service and Pay Book'.

Trade on Enlistment: Clerk.
Enlisted at Perth on 1.3.40
For the: Territorial Army

Complexion: Fresh
Hair: Black

Here's his prisoner-of-war documents, spanning his three-and-a-half-year incarceration from '42 to '45. There's the 'reassurance' card sent to family, in this case to Mrs J. Patterson (his mum), the kind of thing you only ever see in London's Imperial War Museum.

From: J Patterson
Nationality: Scotch
Rank: Pte
Camp: No.2 Penn Camp Thailand

There's an official stamp on the address side, 'PASSED P.W 8199', on the other side an update on his conditions, pre-printed sentences with blank spaces to be filled in by officials (in capitals) or sentences to be left or scored out by officials. It's all propaganda: my dad, like all prisoners, was starved to near death while working on the infamous Thai-Burma Death Railway.

Imperial Japanese Army
I am interned in THAILAND
My health is excellent
~~I am ill in hospital~~
I am working for pay
~~I am not working~~
Please see that FAMILY is taken care
My love to you

James [his real signature]

There's his field medical card, detailing the life-threatening diseases which killed so many of his fellow prisoners.

Malaria ST Five Attacks BT 3 Attacks } Last attack
August 1945
Diarrhoea Occasional attacks since August 1943
Beri 1942 Neuritis + Cardiac
Tonsillitis 1942 Dipheritie
Examination Dental treatment not regained
Weight 11 st 6 lb
Date: 13/10/45

It's a miracle he survived. One hundred thousand men who worked on the railway didn't. So, of course, it's a miracle I got to be here at all. I'd often thought about him, in fact, through the worst of my treatment months. Compared to what my father endured, for three and half years, and the recovery years afterwards? *Come on.* This is a life blip, an inconvenience, a grimly tedious and painful development I must see through to the end with as much patience as I can muster. If I was 'strong' in any way, it was surely partly because of what happened to my staggeringly stoic, never complaining dad – my template for powering through. 'Still waters,' as Mum always said about him, 'run deep.'

There are photos here of the first years of their marriage. Oh my. *What style.* They're walking down a high street, the black-and-white photo as if ripped from the reel of a late forties Hollywood movie, my mum, permed hair swept back, chisel-cheekboned, wearing little round glasses, a light flannel overcoat belted at the waist. A classic forties handbag in one hand, her other is linked through my dad's arm, one hand in his pocket.

My oh my, he is handsome. Tall, raven-haired, a smile on his clean-shaven face, wearing a light, canvas jacket with matching tie over a white, button-down collared shirt, above dark, gentleman's trousers. They couldn't be more striking if they were Clark Gable and Carole Lombard themselves. No kids as yet, and with nine years between them, she must still be the teenager who nursed him back to life, Dad maybe twenty-eight, an elegant man wearing what could well be his Sunday best.

Here they are now in their sociable years, in a club with buddies I don't know, laughing, Dad now with a fifties pencil moustache, Mum with horn-rimmed glasses, a table full of beer, wine and whisky glasses. Here they are in another club, Mum wearing a rollneck, knee-length sixties dress, with her sister, my Aunty Isa, and Uncle Alan, my dad's pencil moustache now slightly thicker, a table hosting pints and half pints, with whisky chasers. It's years before whatever demon turned up in the seventies and changed my mum into an abusive screaming stranger until the demon disappeared and she'd metamorphose back into the dedicated nurse and domestic presence who always took care of everyone. I'm reminded as I sift, transfixed, through the photos strewn over my biggest big sister's dining table, of an exchange between myself and Dad, when I was fifteen, and thought I knew what I was talking about.

'You don't have to put up with this, Dad. Why don't you just leave her?'

'Ach, ma wee pal,' he reassured, an arm around my shoulder. 'You don't know the woman I married.'

Well, here she is right now: standing with my dad, his arm around her, outside what might be their first home in the countryside, Dad wearing a brooding black suit, Mum in a sort of forces' sweetheart uniform of black pleated skirt, white shirt, black tie and fitted cardigan; hanging out of the window of the same house, laughing, with a woman I don't know; in a photobooth, smiling, the gap between her two front teeth clearly visible, wearing a boxy, shoulder-padded early fifties jacket; the pair of them in deckchairs, fully clothed, no doubt frozen somewhere on the blustery east coast of Scotland; in her nurse uniform, dancing, being given some kind of award; with my dad in the home I grew up in, enveloped in each other's arms. Most of these photos I've never seen before. The woman I didn't know. Right there. After all these years.

And there *we* are in London in 1996, the only time she ever came to visit, when Jackie brought her down, seven years after the death of my dad, eight years before her own. She was sixty-six but seemed eighty-six, now a benign, fragile figure, a few years clean from the booze. We had a blast, boggling at the crown jewels and giggling all the way through Madame Tussauds. I'm so glad she made that trip. She wrote in her diary at home afterwards, open for all to see: 'I feel like I've been all the way around the universe.'

Liz slides over another unexpected parcel, a tied-up collection of letters. Can these be . . . love letters? Oh lord, *they are*. Love letters written by my dad to my mum. Between the post-hospital recovery years and the altar. Jackie won't look: 'Too private.' Liz has already looked. 'Just a little look.' I, too, will have a little look.

Dear Rita...

Momentarily, I stop breathing. In his familiar, elegant handwriting he starts off saying he's well and he misses her . . . and I won't read any more, give him, and her, back their privacy. But I'm nosy. I'd just like to see how he signed himself off. I turn the final page.

Your lover for life,
Jimmy

Tears spring immediately. Of course they do. It's so unexpected, so intimate, so *committed*. The source of my own life, right there, almost two decades before I was born. He called himself *Jimmy*. He was James, Jim very occasionally, but never Jimmy in all the years I knew him. But he was Jimmy once. When these people were nothing to do with me. Before they had four other children before me. I tie the letters back up again and see a chin-wobbling glance from Liz.

There's one final, unexpected memento. A photocopy of a newspaper cutting from Tuesday 24 June 1980, detailing the winners of a Perth Rotary Club essay competition, a tiny arrow pointing to the luminously peroxide head of the fifteen-year-old schoolgirl about to be booted out of every pub and club in Perth (apart from the Wheel Inn). Mum had kept it all these years. There must have been some sense of pride after all. All I remembered, from those bad old days, was the shame she voiced over my post-punk hair, the way she apologised to my English teacher for the way I looked, how she only ever described me to my face as a monster from outer space. Poor Mum, I now think. A widow at fifty-nine. Whose own father took his own life. Who lost three brothers throughout her younger life: one in a childhood cycling accident, one in the Second World War and one she nursed in a psychiatric hospital for the last years of his life, a brilliant academic and severe schizophrenic who'd been given a then-brutal treatment, a lobotomy, with the same catatonic outcome as Jack Nicholson's character in *One Flew Over The Cuckoo's Nest*. How punishingly sad, I now feel, that she was left with no friends by her sixties. That she endured prison for three long months in 1995, caught in the grip of an addiction I didn't understand, not then, and only wish I could've helped her with, somehow, had I been significantly more grown-up. But I wasn't. Only rock bottom saved her, as is so often the way with addicts.

A memory floats in. We're in her living room, the year before she died, a white-haired seventy-three-year-old, still smoking her Benson & Hedges, between puffs on the now permanent oxygen nebuliser at her feet.

How old d'you feel on the inside, Mum?

'Twenty-one!' she announced, without hesitation.

I didn't believe her for a second; she seemed so old and frail. But that was all on the outside. At twenty-one she was a busy, stylish, thrilled new mum of three, her husband – as these photos and letters so clearly attest – a devoted, strikingly handsome, exquisitely tailored six-footer who'd give Cary Grant a run for his movie-star money. Maybe, that day in her living room, she truly felt she was, on the inside, despite everything, that same old girl after all.

Me? I was now on my way to Perth. Meeting up with Ali for the first time since the Gerry Cinnamon knees-up in Aberdeen, in the weeks I was certain I was dying. The person who always reminds me of the girl I used to be.

37

WHEN I'M 64

It's been two years and four months since we last saw each other in real life, the longest continuous physical absence since we were five years old. Stepping down from the train at Perth station, with Simon, there she is, standing on the platform, idiotic grin beaming across her face. She charges towards me, arms stretched out like an albatross, as ever, smelling of Estée Lauder's 'Youth Dew', as ever, and it feels like ten minutes since I last saw her, as ever.

She looks quizzically at my hair, possibly wondering what her hundred-pound donation to the £170 hairdo robbery actually bought me, the subtle blonde highlights long faded, the threadbare style still growing out into a floppy fringed approximation of the hairdo David Beckham was 'sporting' in 1998.

'What?' I grin. 'Is it hellish!?'

'No ... it's good. I just thought it would be ... blonder!'

Two hours later we're in the pub. And absolutely nothing whatsoever has changed. Or has it?

We're staying with Ali for almost a week in her flat in Perth, bought in the wake of her mum's death in 2017. It's three days after my fifty-seventh birthday and she wants to take me out for lunch but before that she, too, has the old photos out, alongside her priceless teenage diaries, causing rib-cracking mirth and the exclamation in unison, 'We were never in!' (Simon, understandably, has gone out, leaving us to it.) She's been sorting through her mum's belongings and her own memorabilia for months, has hundreds of photos still in their Snappy Snaps packets, the living-room floor strewn with the physical evidence of so much of the life we've shared. The sound of Bon Jovi's 'Livin' On A Prayer' undulates out from the TV screen, set to Radio 2.

She has photos of every holiday we've ever been on as adults, starting with a Club 18–30 holiday in 1986, the year we turned twenty-one, in Ibiza, where I'm mostly sporting a black, Killing Joke promotional army shirt (pinched from the *Smash Hits* competitions room), black-and-white leggings and vertical hair, conspicuously staying out of the sun. I pick one up from that holiday, of us and a ginger-haired young man I was attempting to pursue.

'And he locked himself in the toilet to get away from you,' she delightedly reminds me.

There are photos of the coastal tour we took with Jill in 1985 to the south of England, where we broke into the locked conservatory of our B&B through a window so we could watch *Live Aid* on TV. Three likely lads we'd befriended in a pub joined us (from Paisley near Glasgow), one of whom, unwilling to skulk through the house as we did (via the window) to use the loo, hung up a large plastic bag on the door and peed in there instead. This became known as The Bag O' Pish.

There's The Four of Us on various skiing holidays, back in the late eighties.

'Look how glamorous everybody else is,' she cringes. 'And we look like blokes! Butch lesbians quite frankly.'

Among the photos, there's a letter she wrote to her mum, from Sydney, in June 1991.

Sylv got a phone call from her mum who said that she was going to stay off the drink this time but we've heard that one many times, so Sylv is not that hopeful. I sent her a handout on how to cope with the psychological problems children develop after a life with an alcoholic so she said that was useful, but Sylv's a lot more strong about it nowadays.

'The drink was definitely never any good for her,' muses Ali, 'but she retained her personality, Sylv. Remember that time I came round for T In The Park and she said what she always said, "I wouldn't walk five yards to hear any of it!" And, "I've heard better on a berry field." She was really funny.'

We leaf some more while, in the background, a Radio 2 news bulletin brings the latest developments from Ukraine, which includes the words 'World War III'. I feel heartbroken for the young today, bombarded with so much horror on their twenty-four-hour screens. Throughout these old photos and diaries, I see only the things you're supposed to be bombarded with as kids: teenage romantic turmoil, parental flashpoints, music, pubs, clothes, exams, sport, dancing, laughing (even in the face of family alcoholism).

'It seems to me,' I say to her, 'looking at all this, despite everything, we were happy kids, weren't we?'

'Oh, absolutely!'

'A case of, "Give us all the adventures this town can give us!"'

'We were making up our own rules. Definitely.'

'When you look over your diaries and see your handwriting, d'you still feel like the same person?'

'Oh God, yes. There's still a complete juvenile twerp in there.'

'D'you think we all do pretty much stay the same?'

'I think so. *Ish*. I think some people change and maybe not really for the better. I think they want to change because they want to park all that, the way they were. Which I think is mad. Because that's what makes you the person that you are. I probably am still very juvenile compared to a lot of my peers. Because I find things so funny in a really ... *stupid way*. It's like in *Mamma Mia*, when Donna's talking about money and the hotel falling apart and never having fun and Tanya says, "Whatever happened to our Donna, life and soul of the party?" And Donna says, "I grew up." And Tanya says, "Well, grow back down again!" A great line. Why do people grow up and turn into boring bastards? Seriously. I mean, obviously and clearly, you've got to be responsible if you've *got* responsibilities, like kids! And a job you want to keep! And a home. You can't be an *idiot*. There's a lot of things I would do diff ... or would I? If you did things differently you wouldn't have the life you have now.'

We remember the times we fell out. Of course we fell out. All friends fall out. But it was never for very long.

'Remember the Holland Park wedding?' she chortles, of the swanky ceremony I took her to in the late eighties while down on a London visit. 'You wanted to go for another drink, I think. And I thought you'd had enough! We'd befriended a couple of gay guys, cadging fags off them and they ran out. So you said, "Don't worry, I'll phone a taxi to go and get us some more!" And you *did*. You phoned an Addison Lee on the *Smash Hits* account, got the driver to buy twenty smokes, and reimbursed him when he got there.' On the way home, she reminds me, I went into one of the default settings of my younger self, a mindset where I was prone to shouting, 'I am thoroughly disapproved of!' this time adding, 'You've never cared about me!' while pounding dramatically at my chest.

'Then, back home, you thought you would be nice and made me toast. I was unconscious in bed so you threw the toast all about my head,' she hoots. 'I got up in the morning, covered in toast and said, "Are we going to Brighton, then?" And you just went, "Aye, let's go to Brighton."'

'Do you feel old?'

'No.'

'Neither do I.'

'I *really* don't. That's what I was thinking the other day when I came out the shower. Fuck's sake I'm nearly sixty. *Me!?* It's *weird*. I think about retirement and think, well, what am I gonna do now? Wait to die?

'There's three big theories of ageing and retirement specifically. One: disengagement. You disengage from life, sit in the house and wait to die. Which my dad clearly did. As soon as he retired at sixty-five. "Oh, I'm no' long for this world, hen." And he lived for another twenty-four years. Two: continuity. You continue to live the way you always have. Three: activity. You become *more* active. But your body is not gonna keep up with your head and the things you want to do. That's what I think I'll struggle with. The minute I can't wipe my own backside? Blue pill.'

She surveys the living-room floor scattered with images of old friends, some of whom are gone already.

'That's another thing about lifelong friendship,' she notes. 'By the time my dad got to eighty-nine there was nobody left for him. All his mates were dead. He was always at the crem [crematorium]. People say, you've got your children, you've so much to live for. But your children have their own lives and grandchildren are even more removed. When you've lost your crew, you've lost your crew. You've lost a lot of *you*. Doesn't matter how many bairns you've got. Because they're a different generation with different *everything*. They're not your *pals*.'

'Before I knew how bad, or how not bad things were for me, for three weeks I thought I was dying. I was *convinced* I was going to die.'

'Well, of course you thought that!'

'Did you think that? Even though you were saying I would be all right?'

'When you went septic, that was fucking close, Sylv. I was really upset after that. I know how bad that is, I used to lecture in it. I thought, Did they get the antibiotics into you quick enough? That's why you were in isolation, hooked up. I was so pissed off at myself because I should've known. You said the mouth was bad, I should've made you go in! I was very scared, that's why I was on you all the time, "What's your white cell count today?" And then it happened again!'

'But if I'd been diagnosed three months later? Because of Covid I might have had no treatment whatsoever and be dead right now.'

'Yep. If you were gonna get it, that was the time! It was crazy in Aberdeen. They were still apparently treating cancer but the diagnostics were the problem. For the first time in two years I had no patients in. Where are all the folk with strokes? Fifteen patients I had in a thirty-four-bed ward. I've never had so many staff in my life. All the services shut down. It was messed up. I hope they learn ... if there's a next time.'

'D'you think I'm still the same old girl I used to be? Or something different?'

'I think you are. You never change. Folk say that about you: Sylv's never changed. And why should you?'

'Well, in some ways I think I've needed to, for my own sanity and everyone else's! In the olden days I was messy a lot of the time ...'

'Well, you're not as hallirackit as you used to be!'

'Hallirackit?'

'Off yer head! Crazy and chaotic and acting like an idiot!'

She's now cackling even louder, about watching old episodes of *Absolutely Fabulous* with her daughters when they were young.

'The kids always used to say Patsy was like you.'

'Oh, were I so glamorous!'

'That episode when she smoked the entire kitchen. That's what you used to do! Put that in yer book! Falling asleep in the bed with the fag in your hand. The amount of times I used to take that out of your paw ...'

'At least it wasn't still in my mouth and burnt my face!'

'Remember you burnt the pillow at T's in Ireland?'

She's talking about a nineties' boyfriend, 'T', whose family were a very gracious, and very religious, middle-class Irish family.

'Did I!?'

'Yes! You went to his folks' house in Ireland and, apart from the fact you couldn't flush the johnny down the toilet ...'

'*What?* Oh, stop!'

'You managed to burn the bed and the pillowcase! In his parents' spare room. Because you went to sleep with a fag in your mouth. D'you not remember that? You told me that!'

'I've told you far too much!'

'Well, there you go, that's pals for you.'

We calm down, stick the kettle on and get ourselves ready for the birthday meal in a new, swish restaurant in Perth. We're a long way, now, from saved-up school dinner money and single snouts from the ice-cream van outside school. It's just past midday on a bright spring morning in 2022, almost one year on from the end of my eighteen months of toxic treatments for breast cancer. And now, Ali tells me something she's never told me before. It's not been a secret, she assures me, it was just all so long ago. Ali herself has had cancer. *Twice.*

'WHAT THE HELL ARE YOU TALKING ABOUT!?'

At nine years old she was in hospital for weeks, for what I've always believed was a burst appendix.

'It never did burst,' she tells me today. 'They got to it beforehand. The doc pressed on my abdomen and I hit the roof. "We're getting her in today, that's close to bursting."

'They operated that day. And that's when they found it. They got the appendix out, accompanied by a two-inch tumour and some of the bowel. I was at the hospital every month for a year afterwards, for tests, to make sure it hadn't come back.'

'I don't remember *any* of that. You certainly didn't whinge about it or even mention it was cancer. Is that because it was pretty much a taboo word back then?'

'It's because I didn't know about it myself until years later! My folks didn't tell me, they didn't want to scare me. I found out when I went into healthcare. It had always bothered me, why I was always going for check-ups. Ev had her appendix out and she was in and out in two days, no follow-ups, tiny scar. My scar was massive. So I asked to go through my medical records and there it was. So at the time I thought it was normal, just something I had to do – go to Edinburgh every month. I remember Mum saying the surgeon didn't know if he'd have to operate on the bowel again. And if so I would've had a bag. A fucking colostomy bag. Cheers! That would've been attractive wouldn't it? That would've curtailed my shagging somewhat. Heheheh!'

'That could so very easily have spread everywhere and you would be dead.'

'Very easily. D'you not remember when I couldn't go to the toilet?'

'No!'

'That's why I felt so bad for you when you had your . . . *situation*. Constipation on that level, there is nothing worse! And it *can* kill you. I used to pass things that size [holds hands out as if fondling a cabbage]. It wasn't medication; the tumour was interrupting the bowel. I was like that for years. We would go to the toilet and you'd be waiting for me for ages.'

'I can't believe you could've been dead at nine, ten years old. No you round-the-corner any more. What the hell would I have done? None of *this*, in all these photos and diaries, would've happened. It's just like *It's A Wonderful Life*. It's true!'

'It *is* true.'

She then tells me about the second time, aged twenty-seven, when she lived in Jersey, with her soon-to-be-husband Billy.

'There were cell changes,' she says, matter-of-factly. 'I went to see about it because of painful sex. They did a biopsy and there were pre-cancerous cells. Then they did a colposcopy, I had everything up there but the kitchen sink. I felt *raped*. They cut a section out and lasered it, got rid of it. It was horrific – not that painful; it was the violation. There was a camera up there, I could see my cervix on the screen. I thought I was never gonna be able to have kids. But it cleared up really well. I had smears every year for four years after that and paid for one at five years, I was still so freaked out.'

No wonder, then, during that rainy car journey from Aberdeen to Stonehaven in November 2019, talking about *Beaches*, she said she always thought it would be her.

'Why didn't you tell me at the time? You didn't have to face all that on your own.'

'To be perfectly honest I was mad in the head at the time! I was being bullied at work, hated the place, wanted to get back to Scotland and I didn't think it was all that big a deal. It wasn't full-blown, it was caught so early. I was more concerned about my mental health!'

'Does it hang over you in any way, the thought of it coming back?'

'It sits there. It sits there, at the back.'

'Like it will do with me, now.'

'It sits there at the back, Sylv. And if anything does go wrong or if anything feels different, for a fleeting moment you always think it's that. *Back*. You just *do*. I *thoroughly* expect to die of cancer, I'm sure it will come back at some point. One day. But it's not *to*day. So get yer eyebrows on. And let's go for a nice birthday meal . . . and a cocktail!'

38

I SHOULD BE SO LUCKY

During the lockdown months of spring 2021, my nature-punk hero Chris Packham created a solo BBC show called *The Walk That Made Me*, a deeply personal re-enactment of the journey in the Hampshire countryside which defined his childhood and informed the poetic, uncompromising, luminously passionate naturalist he is today.

Towards the end of this masterful, moving piece of broadcasting, he detailed his adolescent struggles with Asperger's syndrome, a young man skittering on the edge of suicide, for whom nature became a lifelong saviour. He surveyed the panoramic, vividly green scenes around the Iron Age fort of St Catherine's Hill, a drone panning out dramatically overhead.

'Those meadows were my playground,' he observed, 'where I came to skip and run and search and learn and escape and survive. Those meadows shaped, and probably saved, my life. My dad is eighty-seven, he's had hip replacements, cataracts, I won't go into his full medical history because he'll think that's private but one thing's for sure. He's not coming up St Catherine's Hill any more. [Audible sigh] The place he led me so many times, he couldn't get up here and I couldn't carry him. After all the times he pushed, pulled, dragged, cajoled and encouraged me up here, he's never going to see the world from the top of this hill again. It's a shame. You've got to push back, *all* the time. You've got to live for every moment. You just can't *count* on tomorrow. Because the day will come when *I* won't be able to climb to the top of St Catherine's Hill. And I don't know when that day is gonna be. I don't know whether this is my last summit attempt on this fabulous old hill fort.'

He then read the final verse from Dylan Thomas' 1951 masterpiece, 'Do Not Go Gentle Into That Good Night', with its deathless final words:

Rage ... rage ... against the dying of the light.

The broadcast ended and a simple message appeared on screen: 'In memory of Colin Harold Packham who recently passed away, 1933–2021'.

Ali drives us into the countryside for a walk through The Hermitage, the ancient forest in Dunkeld we've been walking through since we were kids.

There's nowhere on Earth quite like The Hermitage, where fallen autumn leaves are permanently visible underfoot, turning the topsoil of the earthen pathways a luminous purply-pink and where young, two-foot trees in springtime still haven't dropped, somehow, their burnished, russet leaves. It's where the surface of monolithic boulders and the trunks and branches of two-hundred-foot tall Douglas fir trees are swathed in vivid green moss, transforming the landscape into a fluorescent forest of lush-green fuzzy felt. It's *so* vivid, *so* colourful, it vibrates the very air. We wander to the waterfall at its centre, the Black Linn Falls, where a thundering, bouncing deluge throws up a fine, cold water spray.

'This is where my ashes are going!' shouts Ali, breezily, as the torrents plunge over prehistoric, furry green rocks. 'Billy's are going into the sea at Stonehaven so we'll maybe meet up somewhere in the ocean. The girls know all about it.'

Ali's ashes. Blimey. Never thought about Ali's ashes before. But she will be ashes one day. As we all will. We drive back to Perth through the village of Luncarty, where my movie-star mum and dad lived back in the fifties and early sixties, where my four siblings grew up before the move to Perth in 1969. This is where my mum, dad and brother Ronnie are now all buried, in the same graveyard plot, all of them ashes now.

We drive past our old Perth homes, through the streets we walked and cycled and pogo-sticked, before boys and clothes and fags and booze and music barged in and altered reality for ever. We drive past the South Inch and the daffodils are out, spring's very own trumpeters, platoons of them parping out the good news: everything's coming back to life. Tonight, we're going to a memorial party, for someone we apparently knew at school, who neither of us remember. But our old pal Rimmy knew her well and insists we'll be welcome. She was one year younger than us and died of breast cancer last year, aged fifty-five.

Every perspective-changing cliché you could ever imagine about surviving a life-threatening illness is almost laughably true, and certainly laughably simple. When you believe you're about to die, the important things in life step out from the maelstrom of everyday reality and line up in clear sight, in fresh, intensely vibrant colours, while the other stuff fades to grey. The things, of course, that were there all along.

Back in 2016 I had my first book published, ostensibly about thirty years in music journalism and its decline into obsolescence. It was only during the writing, though, that the subtext came to light: I'd been searching for the Meaning of Life through the dubious source of a three-decades-long, zigzagging conga line of bonkers pop stars and chaotic rock'n'roll reprobates. The answer, I concluded, lay somewhere between two pronouncements in two different decades, from glitter-frocked sixties' soul diva Diana Ross in 1986 and blarney-tongued rock'n'roll Pope-botherer Bono in 2000.

The fabulous Miss Ross leaned in towards me with a very-important-pronouncement.

'Can I just tell you the truth here?' she glimmered, promisingly. 'Money does *not* bring you happiness. The things that really bring happiness don't require it. Like good friends and family. Going for a picnic. Going on a long walk. Relationships. Dancing or reading a good book. Watching a daffodil grow.'

Bono, fourteen years later, was musing on the title of U2's latest album, *All That You Can't Leave Behind*, when his very-important-pronouncement seemed to me, at the time, as true a summation of the Meaning Of It All as I'd ever heard. The title, he intoned Bono-ly, was inspired by a passage from the Scriptures, about 'the fire you pass through and all the straw and wood and bollocks is burned away and you're left with the eternal things, like friendship and like love and like laughter.'

All of that was decades before cancer. And before my mother's death, and Gavin's death and three miscarriages and the deaths of more old friends and acquaintances and heroes and the death, now, of every one of the parents of The Four of Us. And it's simply *more* true, and increasingly true, with each day I stay alive.

Sometimes I'll ponder the nature of happiness through the thoughts of the ancient thinkers, the ones we acknowledge as the masters of eternal wisdom.

'Sorrow can be alleviated,' mused thirteenth-century Italian friar philosopher Thomas Aquinas, 'by good sleep, a bath and a glass of wine.'

Which makes me smile, recalling those gruelling months of no sleep and the puddle bath and the zero booze. There, I inwardly nod, I *knew* it. Everything else is the people you love, a decent home, a sense of safety, some kind of purpose (work or otherwise), community connections, the natural world, not being broke and good-enough health, both physical and mental. But mostly it's the people you love. Or, as the prodigiously gifted Barry Gibb put it in a 2020 Bee Gees documentary, reflecting on having sold 220 million albums against the loss of his three younger brothers, 'I'd rather have them all back and no hits.'

Believing I was going to die has changed me, yes, but so has simply being this age, as it surely will for anyone should they reach these still bafflingly 'seasoned' years. I've learned I have even more patience than I thought I had, even more acceptance of feeling hideously awful month after month than I ever thought I would. Because when you have no choice, you just *do*. The older you become, the more life will hurl its bricks through the window of your reality and the more astonished you will be at just how much shock, grief, horror, sadness, turmoil and the full spectrum of the Big Stuff it turns out you can tolerate, after all. And maybe even transcend.

I feel as physically well as I've ever felt – in fact *better* than I have in years, what with the constant walking and the yoga and the sacking off the vape and the nutritious food cooked in copper-bottomed pans in the sparkling Kitchen of Joy.

For twenty-four months I was stabbed, punctured, gouged, sliced, diced, stapled, frozen, fevered, poisoned, syphoned and had every cell of my body incinerated – a bit, perhaps, like a pyrolytic self-cleaning oven. The result? Protocol today means you're never told you are 'cancer-free'. So I am what they call NED, the latest tests having determined there is No Evidence of Disease. Which also makes me smile – where I'm from, a 'ned' is a cap-sleeve-T-shirted football hooligan out on the lash, intent on a taxi-rank punch-up. But this NED I will happily be.

I'm not in denial: I know this thing can come back. So, I either live a shadowy half-life in fear and diminish the time I have left. Or, I spring out of bed every day like Spike Milligan and shout, 'Hooray, another day!' I don't feel collared, either, by the random icy fingers of bad luck. On the contrary, I've never felt so lucky in my life. Cancer still kills people, every second of every day. It didn't kill me, not this time. Perhaps not ever.

All of us at some point, without exception, will endure severely traumatic life events and it's those events, more than any others, which will let us know just how fragile and fleeting our lives, and all life, truly is. Wandering past the Marie Curie charity shop in Perth, a quote on a sign in the window sprang out to greet me. 'Mostly it is loss which teaches us about the worth of things' – Arthur Schopenhauer.

Science, meanwhile, marches on. There are clinical trials ongoing for cancer vaccines, research creating the possibility, at last, of a cancer-free future. Here in the present, the Cancer Research UK stats are phenomenally encouraging: state-of-the-art, targeted treatments evolve every year, giving us years more than we would've had, even ten years ago. *Lucky.* Breast cancer survival has almost doubled in the UK in the last forty years, since I was a teenager, from 40 to 78 per cent. *Lucky.* Seventy-five per cent of breast cancer patients – *three out of four of us* – live for *at least* another ten years. And if you're young enough, for several decades more. *Lucky.*

It's not going away any time soon: one in seven women in the UK (and globally) will be diagnosed with breast cancer sometime in their lives, but the majority will survive. Less than a quarter of the 55,000 women still diagnosed every year will die from it. We need to know that. I wish I'd known that back in the winter of 2019 when the word cancer, to my ears, meant certain, imminent death. I'd no idea, back then, that this thing would probably not kill me. At least, not yet.

I think back, now, to the conversation with fellow survivor Kylie and understand, much more, what she meant in 2007 by her 'changed perspective', for the better.

'Yes,' she nodded, 'because now and then I will think, God, I might not even be here. I could've just ignored it. And it could be a very different story. That's why organisations bang on; people think it's never gonna happen to them, they think, Oh, I can't be bothered going to the doctor's, and we all need to be reminded of common sense.'

By 2019, the year of her glorious Glastonbury performance, the year after she turned fifty, she was contemplating whether she could keep touring at sixty.

'I'd be happy just to be sixty, regardless!' she laughed. 'Just to *be* here is amazing. If my showbiz hips and knees can keep doing it, then we'll be good.'

She sounded to me, at fifty-one, like she'd reached a new level of creative and personal fulfilment, was maybe even at peace with herself, at last?

'Definitely,' she said, emphatically. 'Without a doubt, this is the best place I've ever been in my life. Yes. *Oof.* Takes a minute to get there, doesn't it?'

Yes, Ms Minogue, *it does*.

Sarah Harding, the celebrated Girls Aloud party girl, was one of the tragically unfortunate ones. Fatally, she stalled over getting herself checked because of Covid, was honest enough to say in public she'd used the lockdown restrictions 'as an excuse not to face up to the fact that something was very wrong'. She died on 5 September 2021, aged just thirty-nine. She made it known she wants no other woman to make her deadly mistake and all we cancer survivors, from now on, will reinforce her legacy. Where she was diagnosed too late, in the wrong year (2020), I was diagnosed early enough, in a right one (2019), just eight short months apart, one victim and one survivor of the lottery of life.

Part of her legacy, too, is the further embedding of the word 'cancer' into mainstream conversation, a torchlight of truth now regularly shone into needlessly shadowy corners by a spectrum of public figures. From BBC news presenter Victoria Derbyshire's breast cancer reflections in the *Celebrity* jungle in 2020, to Sky Sports presenter Jacquie Beltrao's regular tweets on her recurring breast cancer through 2021, to a bowel cancer diagnosis for *First Dates'* barman Merlin Griffiths in autumn 2021 and Julia Bradbury's much-admired ITV documentary *Breast Cancer And Me* in April 2022. Watching the latter, for me, was a bittersweet experience. Julia, seated on her bed, courageously and unselfconsciously allowed cameras to film the moment she saw her breast reconstruction for the first time.

'Bloody hell!' I shrieked out loud, freeze-framing the moment to fully take in the vision of a breast implant she was dismayed to find 'lumpy', while I could barely tell which one was which; an astounding feat of surgical wizardry. With apologies to the fabulous Julia, I clearly had implant envy, memories flashing back of the space hopper, the Tunnock's teacake and the half-eaten octopus head.

But that spring/summer of 2022 also brought profound gratitude once more, as we witnessed the deaths of two gallingly young public figures. Tom Parker from boyband The Wanted, from a brain tumour at the age of thirty-three. And the most high-profile living-with-cancer patient in British history, Dame Deborah James, a.k.a. BowelBabe, gone at just forty. She left an immortal legacy: not only the seven million pounds she raised for cancer charities, but her indelible smile and her final message for the millions she inspired (and the countless lives she'd already saved). 'Find a life worth enjoying; take risks; love deeply; have no regrets; and always, always have rebellious hope.'

Her name was Karen. Rimmy knew her long after we'd moved away from Perth, a music person, a dancer, and the DJ chosen for her memorial party is the DJ from the Banana Club, when I was seventeen years old: my then-boyfriend and musical mentor John McKeand.

Walking into Perth's Civil Service Club, an old-school civic hall, a beaming Rimmy approaches. 'There's a free bar!' he grins. Blimey, a free drink or two before it runs out, everyone thinks.

It's a free bar *all night long*.

Up on stage there's John, busy on the wheels o' steel. 'This is so weird!' I yelp to Simon, hands flying onto my face, John blasting out the Style Council's 'Speak Like A Child'. I jump up on stage, throw my arms around his startled shoulders and start babbling on about the Spotify playlists he started during lockdown which I played on the sunny balcony in the early days of Covid and my double imprisonment as an NHS 'vulnerable'.

A piper appears at the door, someone shouts out to follow him, everyone grabs their glass and heads outdoors where the piper now parps a triumphant 'Flower Of Scotland'. From somewhere nearby in the inky darkness a firework flares upwards and explodes overhead, a falling galaxy of sparkles disintegrating under starry Scottish skies. Then, another one. Then, a spontaneous, heartfelt and emotionally powerful round of clattering applause. These fireworks, we're now told, were filled with Karen's ashes, the pyrotechnic parting shot so many choose today, her ashes scattered across the sky from where they'll fly and fall throughout the town she grew up in. Someone shouts, laughing, 'Who's next? Barry's next!'

I'm standing next to Rimmy.

'Rim? If this was me, if I *had* died, this would be as good as it would get.'

'If it was me? Lug me in a bin bag and leave me to the dogs. Dinnae put me in the ground! Fuckin' no way, in that cold, dark earth!' He looks around at the assembled, grown men and women hugging each other, everywhere. 'Fuckin' hell, we've all gotta go sometime,' he ponders. 'Somehow. As long as you keep waking up in the morning.'

'It's getting weird, isn't it?'

'I know.'

We go back inside, onto the dancefloor, and the songs keep coming. The old songs. And it's here, in this communal setting, in this emotionally heightened party atmosphere, that the music from The Olden Days, after all, comes surging back to life, every atom of its original power, every thread of that suddenly no-longer-frayed magic carpet still capable of pan-dimensional flight: 'Do I Love You' by Frank Wilson, 'Cath' by The Bluebells, 'Oblivious' by Aztec Camera, 'This Charming Man' by The Smiths, 'Party Fears Two' by The Associates, 'Into The Valley' by Skids, 'She Is A Belter' by Gerry Cinnamon (the lone contribution tonight from the twenty-first century), 'She Sells Sanctuary' by The Cult, 'Transmission' by Joy Division, 'When You're Young' by The Jam...

Everyone here knows every word of every one of these songs, a colossal communal singsong, just the way Scotland likes it, on a permanently packed dancefloor. A palpable sense of elation is lifting us all off the floor, people's faces bursting with joy, arms forever in the air, delirious with that feeling only familiar music and exuberant dancing can give you – abandon, ecstasy, *freedom*. It's been *years* since I've danced like this, out here in public, not in the kitchen, and with these people especially, each song conjuring a dizzying vision of the young people we all once were, singing and dancing just like this, thirty-five, forty years ago, together. I can see our faces, the clothes we wore, the hair on the heads of the men who no longer have hair.

A man with plenty of hair I've never met before keeps bounding over to me for a dance, huge smile on his face, a tall fella wearing a mod-ish jacket. It's maybe the fourth time we're bouncing around each other when he leans into my face and shouts, in jubilation, 'You're gorgeous!'

What!?

I'm astounded, thrilled – this kind of thing hasn't happened to me for *twenty years*. I tell Ali and she roars with laughter.

'Still got it!' we both bawl, with an extravagant, stinging high five.

The last song has been immaculately chosen: Prince Buster's 'Enjoy Yourself', a song memorably covered by The Specials, and none more fitting for this celebration of a woman I did not know and a life I did not share. This celebration of the euphoria of life itself. It truly could not have been more fitting if it *was* my own funeral. And when I die, I think to myself, I want *this* level of dancing (if you lot aren't off-your-legs by then), and *this* level of drinking (if you've any pancreas left), although you'll be paying for it yourselves, my friends, I could never shoulder a bar tab for the likes of *you*.

'Enjoy yourself!' bawls the crowd of middle-aged revellers, in a slightly tattered old town hall, in a slightly tattered old Scottish city in the spring of 2022, as the bombs rain down on the citizens of Ukraine and there's talk every day of nuclear war, even more than there was back in 1980 when we all first danced to this elevational song.

'Enjoy yourself!' we roar on, as one, '*it's later than you think . . .*'

Back in London some weeks later, myself and Simon are walking downwards through the paths of Alexandra Park, on the way home from Muswell Hill in the newly descended darkness. The lights of the big city stretch out across the horizon, the full span of the iconic skyline clearly visible, distant towering obelisks thrusting upwards through necklace strings of dazzling silvery streetlight. A cluster of building cranes here in the north, the tallest objects in this panoramic view, are geometric shapes lit up by burning red lights, a constellation of dramatic, scarlet suns. Above our heads there's the rare sight, here in the light-polluted city, of the three unmistakeable stars of Orion's Belt, the Girdle of the Celestial Hunter, his starry bow poised and arcing upwards towards the vastness of the universe, where we live, on the lonely planet the cosmological crusader Carl Sagan once so memorably described as 'a mote of dust, suspended in a sunbeam'. I let go of Simon's hand, my arms flying into the air.

'Oh God, I'm gonny miss life when I'm dead!'

And that's all it is, this death thing. You just *think* you'll miss life, but of course you won't. Because you don't miss anything when you're dead. You only miss things when you're alive. So while you are? *Get busy livin'*. If you just can't count on tomorrow, make sure you can count on today.

I know I could be dead, still, in two years' time. In five. In ten. So could you. I could be dead tomorrow if I'm very unlucky. So could you and everyone you know.

But I'm not dead yet. And neither are you.

Lucky us.

THANK YOU

(Turned out to be a wonderful life after all)

BUILDING AND LOAN

You gave this thing legs, a purpose and a road ahead: Kevin 'Agent P' Pocklington (for the belief, and the night of the Dancing Queens); the team at Fleet (Little, Brown); Rhiannon Smith (for the empathy, vision and enormous schnitzels), Amy Perkins (for the guidance and forensics) and Stephanie Melrose (the queen of encouragement).

CLARENCE

Infinite gratitude for the rest of my life (for giving me a rest of my life) to the cancer treatment team at London's Northern Hospital (for the skills, knowledge, kindness, integrity, humanity and good humour. All in a day's work. In a global pandemic.) For legal/privacy reasons I'm unable to name the real hospital, and all names of the staff who treated me have been changed. I sincerely hope, by the time this book comes out, you've all had a massive pay rise.

BEDFORD FALLS

Gigantic 'blub!' to my lifelong friends, for their unflinching support, for their words, deeds, silly things, practical things, delicious things and spectacularly stupid jokes: Leesa Reeve-Daniels, Trish and Bob Darvell, Gillian Best, James Ross, Craig McLean, Tommy the D, Karen McCombie, Gillian

Porter, Tom Sheehan, Andy Prevezer, Rimmy, Bruce Shaw, D. J. and Sarah MacLennan, Siân Pattenden and the generous friends and family of the Hockings in St Albans. Beyond-the-call blubs to Evelyn Hocking (for providing not only support, but the blanket, soup, cake, Easter, Glasto and selfless services as my personal Parker for the 'best' part of a year); Jill Henry (for enough swanky wine and cheese to see me dead from gout instead 'ho' 'ho'); and Ali Doyle (for the advice, vigilance and hairdo, for the diaries, dancing and cackles, and the blaring in my ear not only through all this madness but the previous fifty years. And you thought I was 'seek' *before*…?!)

THE BAILEYS

Commemorative thanks to my parents, James and Rita Patterson (who showed me how to survive). And to my fabulous, inspirational family: Jackie, Liz, Brendon, Sergi, Jenna, Thomas. There's now good stuff on the way for all of us, isn't there? Isn't there!?

320 SYCAMORE

You gave me shelter, sanity and the heat of a man-shaped electric blanket. I gave you some bonnie kitchen tiles. And if you hadn't been there with me through it all (and only you know what 'it all' truly means), I might have died of trauma, starvation and isolation anyway. But you were, and I didn't. 'Simon Goddard, I'll love you till the day I die.'

CREDITS

1 https://www.panmacmillan.com/authors/philippe-auclair/
  cantona/9780230747012
2 *Guardian*, 20 May 2021

p.21, 'Do They Know It's Christmas?'
Words and music by Bob Geldof and Midge Ure © 1984

p.67, 'Perfect Skin'
Words and music by Lloyd Cole © 1984

p.78, '5.15'
Words and music by Pete Townshend © 1973

p.111, *Rocky Balboa*
Directed by Sylvester Stallone, screenplay by Sylvester
Stallone © 2006

p.166, 'Into The Groove'
Words and music by Madonna and Stephen Bray © 1985

p.172, 'Say Something'
Words and music by Kylie Minogue, Jonathan Green, Ash
Howes and Richard Stannard © 2020

p.234, 'Stabbed'
Words by James Allan, music by Ludwig van Beethoven © 2008

p.246, 'You Get What You Give'
Words and music by Gregg Alexander and Rick Nowels © 1998

p.283, 'Enjoy Yourself'
Words by Herb Magidson, music by Carl Sigman © 1949

INTERVIEWS: SOURCE PUBLICATIONS

pp.8, 279, Kylie Minogue: *Q*, December 2007, and Official Press
Biog Interview, 2019

p.24, Jarvis Cocker: *Sky*, November 1995

pp.33, 86, 98–9, 200–1, Tyler James: Interview for *My Amy, The Life We Shared* (Macmillan), 2021

p.88, Jennifer Aniston: *Glamour*, 2011

p.89, Zac Efron: *Glamour*, January 2010

p.89, Madonna: *NME*, March 1998

p.89, Matty Healy: *Q*, November 2018

p.90, Liam Gallagher: *MOJO*, November 2007

p.100, Shaun Ryder: *Sky*, 1995

p.112, Jay Kay: *Sky*, November 1996

p.119, David Beckham: *The Face*, July 2001

p.121, Nicky Wire: *NME*, August 1998

p.176, Spike Milligan: *NME*, 1996

p.182, Nicola Roberts, Girls Aloud: *Observer*, October 2008

p.183, Pete Burns: *Guardian Guide*, April 2003

pp.190–4, Pete Doherty: *The Word*, 2006, and *Q*, 2013

p.201, Amy Winehouse: *The Word*, March 2007

p.247, Lewis Capaldi: *Q*, August 2019

p.248, Debbie Gibson: *Guardian*, November 2021

p.252, Bobby Gillespie: *Q*, June 2019

p.276, Diana Ross: *Smash Hits*, 1986

p.276, Bono: *NME*, October 2000